STO

ATTENTION!
BAR CODE IS LOCA
INSIDE OF BOOK

Y0-ABP-998

DO NOT REMOVE
CARDS FROM POCKET

ALLEN COUNTY PUBLIC LIBRARY

FORT WAYNE, INDIANA 46802

You may return this book to any agency, branch,
or bookmobile of the Allen County Public Library.

DEMCO

STO

ACPL ITEM
DISCARDED

COUNTY PUBLIC LIBRARY

Wolfe, Maxine

Practical pregnancy

2.4.80

2 · 4 · 80

Practical
Pregnancy

Practical Pregnancy

All That's Different in Life Because You're Pregnant

by Maxine Gold Wolfe

& Margot Goldsmith

Foreword by
Martin N. Motew, M.D.
and Jorge A. Valle, M.D.

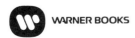

WARNER BOOKS

A Warner Communications Company

Copyright © 1980 by Maxine Gold Wolfe and Margot Goldsmith
All rights reserved.
Warner Books, Inc., 75 Rockefeller Plaza, New York, N.Y. 10019

W A Warner Communications Company

Medical illustrations by David Bruce Wolfe

Fashion illustrations by Ray Skibinski

Distributed in the United States by Random House, Inc., and in
Canada by Random House of Canada, Ltd.
Portions of this book first appeared in *McCall's Working
Mothers Magazine* and *Ms. Magazine.*

Acknowledgments:
J. B. Lippincott Company for Figure 14, "Prenatal Weight Gain
Grid," from *Clinical Obstetrics,* 1953.
The California Department of Health, Maternal and Child Health
Branch, for Table 1, "Daily Food Guide," and Table 2, "Food Groups."
Adapted from *Nutrition During Pregnancy and Lactation, 1975.*
Printed in the United States of America
First Printing: May 1980
10 9 8 7 6 5 4 3 2 1

Library of Congress Cataloging in Publication Data

Wolfe, Maxine Gold.
  Practice pregnancy.

  Bibliography: p.
  Includes index.
  1. Pregnancy. 2. Prenatal care. 3. Childbirth.
I. Goldsmith, Margot, joint author.
RG525.W64   618.2'4   79-22003
ISBN 0-446-51204-4

Book design by Helen Roberts

Foreword

2099087

In the course of my obstetrical practice I can often only sympathize with my pregnant patients when they share their feelings and questions with me. Due to my busy schedule, and perhaps more importantly, due to not knowing what to ask, mothers-to-be don't spend a lot of time asking the practical, nonmedical questions they have about their pregnancies. Of course, that presumes I could answer them with some authority!

What this book provides to the expectant mother and doctor alike is a reference for not only the medical, but also the practical aspects of being pregnant. Most obstetricians can explain to a woman what physical changes she will experience and how to deal with them, but when it comes to an explanation of what maternity clothing is available, or how pregnancy may affect work, or what important questions a woman should be asking her doctor, the conversation usually ends.

The pregnant woman, her partner, and their doctor should have very few unanswered questions after reading this book. The thoroughness of the authors is readily evident, in the extensive topics covered and in the authoritativeness of the information. The authors have painstakingly gathered this accurate information by consulting practicing physicians, lawyers, insurance agents, nurse-midwives, nutritionists, and physiologists, and drawing on the experiences of their own pregnancies.

Having reviewed and read many books on pregnancy, written mostly by doctors, I feel this patient-oriented text is a unique, modern approach to an ageless subject.

There is a definite bias in this book toward informing the pregnant woman of her rights, such as the right to choose her birth attendant and the right to decide where her delivery will take place. Other controversial subjects are approached; the pros and cons of each side are discussed and backed up by facts.

To make sure that all my patients read this book, I plan to give them a copy at their first prenatal visit rather than suggest that they go out and buy it. There is, of course, a distinct advantage to this approach. Patient education leads to healthier pregnant women, who will tolerate the discomforts of pregnancy readily and safely. I also believe that patients who read this book will be a definite threat to the uninformed provider of pregnancy care. This upgrading of patient knowledge and questioning of medical care can undoubtedly benefit our most important product—our children.

Martin N. Motew, M.D., F.A.C.O.G.
Attending
Department of Obstetrics and Gynecology
Michael Reese Hospital
Chicago, Illinois

Clinical Associate Professor
University of Chicago
Pritzker School of Medicine
Department of Obstetrics and Gynecology

In the last twenty years there has been a dramatic improvement in techniques for evaluating fetal and maternal well-being. These techniques have significantly brightened the picture for mothers and babies. Unfortunately, while treating the *problems* of pregnancy, we physicians have often overlooked the *routine needs* of pregnant women. Because of the demands of practice, we do not always provide adequate patient education, or take enough time to encourage patients' questions.

There have been many attempts, by both physicians and lay people, to write informative books on pregnancy. To date, all of these efforts have been less than satisfactory. This book fills the gaps and deficiencies. It offers answers to questions that physicians are often too busy to discuss, and patients are uncomfortable in asking. It dispels many traditionally held misconceptions. By providing pregnant women with information, the book serves not only to educate but to prepare.

Expectant parents and their physicians can be partners. An informed patient can help herself obtain the kind of correct care, which is, after all, the goal of prenatal care. The end result of this partnership will be a happier and healthier pregnancy and a satisfying labor and delivery. I would encourage all pregnant women and their physicians to have a copy of this book close at hand.

Jorge A. Valle, M.D., F.A.C.O.G.
Attending
Department of Obstetrics and Gynecology
Michael Reese Hospital
Chicago, Illinois

Contents

Chapter 4. Common Discomforts and Complications   58

Coping with: Frequent urination. Nausea. Fatigue. Vaginal discharge. Candida albicans. Trichomonas vaginalis. Nonspecific vaginitis. Nosebleeds and stuffy nose. Constipation. Hemorrhoids. Swelling. Excessive salivation. Backache and frontache. Shortness of breath. Leg cramps. Heartburn. Varicose veins. Toxemia (preeclampsia, eclampsia). Ectopic pregnancy. Spontaneous abortion. Multiple pregnancy. Hydatidiform mole. Rh and other blood factors.

Chapter 5. Staying Healthy to Keep Your Baby Healthy   68

Weight gain. Nutritional needs. Vitamins. Dangerous substances in foods. Feeding the newborn. Nutritional needs during lactation. Breast-feeding. Bottle-feeding. Drugs and medications. Alcohol. Nicotine. Caffeine. Marijuana. LSD. Heroin. Aspirin. Tranquilizers. Oral contraceptives. Diuretics. Amphetamines. Antihistamines. Antibiotics. X rays. Radiation. Bibliography.

Chapter 6. The Emotional Side   95

A sense of the future. Reactions. Timing. Marital status. First or subsequent pregnancy. The reactions of others. Getting the news. Worries. Self-image. Preparation. Surroundings. Career concerns. You and your partner. Support systems. Sexuality. Fears and fantasies. Stress. Parents. The extended family. Sibling rivalry.

Chapter 7. Methods of Giving Birth   110

Preparing for birth. Classes. Education. Relaxation techniques. Breathing techniques. Exercises. The partner's role. Teachers: Grantly Dick-Read. Fernand Lamaze. Sheila Kitzinger. Robert A. Bradley. Margaret Gamper. Where to take classes. Cesarean birth. Leboyer method. Further information sources.

Introduction

For nine months, everything changes: your clothing, your doctors, your emotions, and, most of all, your body. You worry about your baby and your health; you wonder where to buy clothes and how much they'll cost. You may be curious about examinations and how often you'll see the doctor. And does insurance cover *everything?*

Pregnancy can be an exhilarating but uncertain time. In very short order you have to find new instincts for coping and develop a foundation for a completely different life-style. You may wonder whether you can adapt to all the changes.

The best thing you can do is get reliable information. Yet, as we discovered when we were pregnant, that information just doesn't exist—at least not in one, accessible place. If we wanted information on job rights, we found we had to contact a knowledgeable lawyer or get transferred from one line to another in federal and state bureaucracies until the right person came to the phone. If we wanted to know about hair care, we had to wait for sporadic newspaper and magazine articles. Maternity clothes shopping? We never did figure out the best way to assemble a wardrobe, and we both wound up buying (all three times) a lot of unnecessary things and wishing we had purchased others.

The popular books on pregnancy were not much help, either. They seemed to discuss only the physiological and emotional aspects of pregnancy and birth. They didn't explore what was so important to us: pregnancy as a nine-month life-style with its own requirements and adjustments. Many books were written by male obstetricians, and we didn't believe they addressed our needs as thinking, feeling, adapting women. We wanted to know about disability insurance, makeup, Lamaze techniques, and sports during pregnancy. We wanted help deciphering insurance policies; we needed tips about comfortable commuting and airplane travel, and information about how other women handled outside jobs.

The result of all the questions we asked was the framework for this book. It was gratifying to discover (by way of lengthy questionnaires we developed and distributed) that other pregnant women were asking the same questions and were frustrated by the lack of answers. So when we set about preparing this guide—a task that became a full year-and-a-half-long project for both of us—we first compiled an exhaustive list of topics and questions that concern expectant mothers today.

Then we went after the answers. We talked with specialists: physicians, nurses, fetal toxicologists, attorneys, job safety experts, childbirth-class instructors, environmental pollution scientists, maternity clothes salespeople, nutritionists, hospital administrators, insurance and employment specialists, geneticists, and several dozen women who had recently been through pregnancies and had a lot to share about their experiences. We asked the airlines about pregnant travelers; we questioned cosmetics companies and federal agencies about product safety. We contacted the major associations most interested in women's health care and women's rights; we went to state and federal government agencies to get the latest data on the laws regarding job rights, disability insurance, and on-the-job hazards. We learned how to assemble safe nursery equipment, how to choose a physician *and* a hospital, and we found out about home birth, genetic testing, nutrition, exercise, and much, much more.

It has been enormously satisfying for us to be able to pull things together, to create a resource for independent, critical-thinking women who want to do more than just "get through" the nine months of pregnancy. In the course of our research we met a woman customer—on her lunch hour—in an expensive maternity shop. She wandered aimlessly around the racks, looking bewildered. We thought of approaching her to ask what the matter was, but at that moment a salesperson came by.

"Can I help you?" the saleswoman asked the bewildered one.

"I'm pregnant," came the reply. "I'm pregnant, and I really don't know what I'm going to need."

She's long since had her baby, but for others who haven't, we hope this book will be useful.

Practical Pregnancy

CHAPTER ONE
If You Think You're Pregnant

Most women are alert to the signs of pregnancy. From the time we have our first sexual encounters, we are tuned into our bodies and notice changes in monthly patterns. Women can catalog and predict bodily changes, and when an unexpected symptom appears—nausea, an unusual or missed period, pelvic congestion—they take notice.

If you think you're pregnant

You want to become pregnant and have stopped using birth control. You've become especially aware of the effect of menstruation on your body, and check periodically for pregnancy symptoms. Intermittent nausea, constipation, tiredness, or nocturia (nok-too'-ree-ah; awakening at night to urinate), although not startling occurrences by themselves, are nevertheless especially notable. You may invest these signs with more meaning than they warrant, but as symptoms mount up, your excitement increases. Whether or not it will be your first pregnancy, it is natural to doubt the reality of the signs and be eager to take a pregnancy test. Before a positive pregnancy test, and before the so-called objective signs a physician or midwife may detect by internal examination, there are changes occurring you will be aware of.

Subjective signs of pregnancy

Called "subjective" because they are not certain tests of pregnancy, these are symptoms women generally first notice themselves. Any of them, alone, may have causes other than pregnancy. The appearance of several, especially if sporadic birth control or no

1

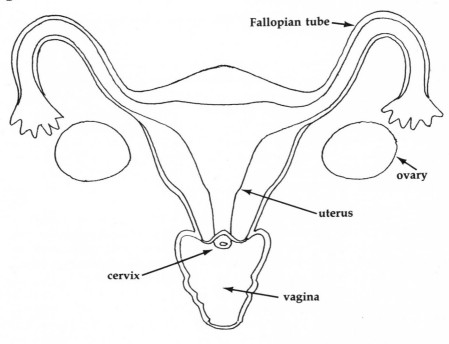

Fig. 1. Female Reproductive System

form of contraception at all is used, strongly indicates that a pregnancy test be performed.

• *Absence of menses, or amenorrhea (a-men-o-ree'-ah).* Menstruation is the monthly loss of the blood-congested uterine lining. In pregnancy this lining is retained as the implantation site for the embryo. If you are regular, miss a period, and suspect conception may have occurred, it's a good idea to go for a pregnancy test. Feminist, low-cost health clinics and home test kits make frequent testing feasible. If you are irregular and seem to be missing periods, you might wait for evidence of other signs of pregnancy. In any case, neither absence nor presence of bleeding is a certain test of pregnancy. Light bleeding may occur during the early months of pregnancy, due to hormonal changes, because of excessive growth of the uterine lining, or simply when the fertilized egg implants in the uterus. Uterine and cervical changes that cause blood loss may occur during pregnancy, too. Absence of bleeding may be caused by illness and worry.

• *Nausea.* Contrary to the myth about its inevitability, only half of the pregnant women in America experience this symptom (the percentage for women outside the United States appears to be lower). Beginning the second week after conception (or four weeks after your last period) you may have wavelike nausea when you wake up in the morning, when you've missed a meal, after you've eaten particular foods, or when you consume alcohol. If you're experiencing prolonged morning queasiness with no illness, you should have a pregnancy test.

• *Congestion in the pelvic region.* A vague ache or feeling of heaviness in the pelvic region may signify pregnancy; unlike premenstrual cramps, the ache is not followed by your period. Many women compare this feeling to the congestion following sexual arousal.

• *Tender breasts.* During pregnancy, the amount of breast tissue and fat actually increases, milk glands grow, and the resultant enlargement and sensitivity may be noticeable in the first few weeks after fertilization. In early pregnancy, you may experience a painful or even tender feeling in your breasts that is like the tingling sensation many women feel before menstruation.

• *Frequent urination, accompanied by an uncomfortable, sluggish urinary sensation.* You may feel like urinating often, yet be surprised at the minimal amount of fluid excreted. By itself, this symptom could also indicate cystitis or other infections.

• *Extreme fatigue.* You may find yourself exhausted and sleepy by midafternoon, barely able to keep up with your young children, or compelled to rest your head on your office desk. You may also need to advance your bedtime by several hours. Pregnancy-related fatigue may be caused by the body's new hormonal patterns. Of course, fatigue alone may not indicate pregnancy but, rather, illness or overexertion.

Confirming your pregnancy

Whether you experience one or many of these subjective signs, if you *believe* you are pregnant, you'll most probably have a pregnancy test.

Where to go for pregnancy tests

Women who don't take home pregnancy tests have a choice about where to be tested. When they suspect they're pregnant, many women have their private obstetricians perform a test. Planned Parenthood and other private family-planning groups and women's health centers offer reduced-cost urine and, occasionally, blood pregnancy tests. City and county boards of health may even provide free pregnancy testing at dozens of accessible locations.

Urine tests

These tests may be done in a doctor's office, a clinic, or a hospital, and most often involve using a sample of urine. This *immunologic* test measures the amount of human chorionic gonadotrophin (ko-ri-on'-ik go-nad-uh-tro'-fin), or HCG—the hormone produced by the developing placenta—in the woman's urine. These tests are 95 to 98 percent accurate if done at least two weeks after the missed period should have begun, or at least forty-one days from the first day of the last menstrual period. These tests can be inaccurate when performed too early—when there is too little HCG present in the urine to produce a positive reaction—and when the pregnancy is abnormal.

Immunologic tests may be done on a slide or in a test tube. On a slide, a small amount of urine is mixed with a substance designed to interact with the HCG hormone; then the slide is slightly agitated for about two minutes. If sufficient HCG is present in the urine, a predictable reaction occurs. Immunologic *tube* tests are based on the same principle but are a bit more accurate than the slide tests. The tube tests usually take about two hours to complete.

The famous "rabbit test"

In our mothers' day, different *biologic* pregnancy tests used laboratory animals, such as rats, frogs, mice, and rabbits, into which the woman's urine was injected. If the animals ovulated, or other signs appeared, the test result was considered positive. Today, the rapidly interpreted and relatively inexpensive (about $15 in a private doctor's office) immunologic tests have generally replaced the more costly biologic tests, which often took two days to complete.

Progesterone test

Another method for determining pregnancy (it is not used much today and is not absolutely safe) involves giving a woman progestin (synthetic progesterone), either orally or by injection, to induce menstruation. Usually, if the woman is not pregnant, bleeding begins a few days after the dosage is stopped. Not only is this procedure less reliable than other methods, but progestin may actually be hazardous to the fetus. Generally, a physician should not administer progestin unless s/he knows you are not pregnant.

Two recent developments in the field of pregnancy testing offer women even faster, more accurate test results, and also the opportunity to have the test in the privacy of their homes.

Blood tests

The radioimmunoassay, or RIA, test can detect pregnancy as early as ten days after conception. This test uses a sample of blood, not urine, with which to detect HCG, and is somewhat more expensive (about $20 to $25 in a private doctor's office) than the urine tests. Depending on the laboratory, results may be available on the same or the next day. The RIA test is good for women who need to know very early if they are pregnant.

Home pregnancy tests

Warner/Chilcott's E.P.T. In-Home Early Pregnancy Test, Acu-Test, and Predictor pregnancy test are immunologic tube tests that can be performed at home on or after the ninth day after the missed period should have begun. The tests take two hours to perform and cost approximately $10 in most drugstores. According to Warner/Chilcott's information, 97 percent of the women who test negative are not pregnant. For those who test negative, E.P.T. literature recommends another test one week later if menstruation has not begun.

Home tests provide women with privacy—only *you* have to know if you're taking a pregnancy test. Also, you can test yourself at your convenience. Even though you need a portion of your first morning urine, you can refrigerate the sample until you are ready to do the test. The cost of home tests is usually less than a private physician charges for a urine test.

You must perform these tests with care in order to get an accurate result. The directions accompanying the home tests are fairly detailed, and each step must be followed precisely. Unreliable test results can occur if the tube is physically disturbed or exposed to sunlight, or if the test is not read after *exactly* two hours.

Accepting the results

If you intend to begin prenatal care with your own physician, s/he will usually accept positive test results from other reliable sources because the findings can be confirmed with a physical examination. On the other hand, if you report a positive test and show none of the uterine or vaginal signs of pregnancy, your physician will probably repeat the urine or blood test.

Why prenatal care?

If you have determined you're pregnant and want to have the baby, it's wisest to begin prenatal care as soon as possible. Some physicians want to see women two weeks after a missed period. In recent years, we've all become aware of how crucial the early days of pregnancy are, and of how drugs, alcohol, and chemicals can adversely affect the fetus. The sooner pregnant women link up with doctors, clinics, or nurse-midwives, the less chance there is of some preventable tragedy's occurring during the first weeks.

Obstetric caretakers can advise women about such vital matters as diet and avoidance of teratogenic (ter-uh-tuh-jen'-ik) (malforming) substances. Through a complete physical exam they can more accurately determine the date of conception and also discuss and evaluate what effect a woman's medical history may have on her pregnancy. This evaluation may include counseling about genetic diseases that can be passed on to the fetus.

Pregnant women have themselves, as well as their babies, to consider. Pregnancy is not an illness, but it does impose stresses on our bodies. The stresses may cause serious health problems for the mother if she is diabetic, anemic, or hypertensive. It is important for the physician or nurse-midwife to obtain *baseline readings* of blood, blood pressure, urine, and other functions to detect any changes occurring later on. On the positive side, regular prenatal care can help eliminate some of the inevitable discomforts of pregnancy and provide answers to the questions women may have.

If you have gone to your own doctor for a pregnancy test, you can begin a program of prenatal care immediately. Some women, as we've mentioned, have the test done at a clinic, board of health, or women's center, then make an appointment to see their doctors for an initial prenatal exam. Keep in mind that obstetric costs are usually a package arrangement—you won't save money by delaying the first visit.

Finding a doctor or nurse-midwife

Women who don't have a doctor or nurse-midwife might try asking friends, contacting local medical societies or health departments, or seeking a referral from another doctor they use. Established health groups, such as Planned Parenthood, childbirth-education groups, and local women's centers, are also good resources for referrals. Pregnancy is such an important and lengthy period that women should shop around and take their time in choosing an obstetric practitioner. Unfortunately, if you're already pregnant, you may feel more pressure to make this choice as quickly as possible. It is essential to see a doctor or nurse-midwife early. But it's also important—whether you're selecting a new doctor or deciding to remain with an old one—to feel comfortable and compatible with the person you'll see a lot of in the coming months.

Most women have a good idea of what kind of personality and expertise their obstetrician or nurse-midwife should have. In addition, they have more or less definite notions of what they desire from the pregnancy and childbirth experience. You have a right—and an obligation to yourself—to discuss these feelings in a polite yet specific way with your doctor. Obstetricians should welcome questions. It's as difficult for them to deal regularly with a patient who doesn't really agree with their methods as it is for you to trust a person who rejects your beliefs.

The first prenatal exam

During your initial prenatal exam, you will give a health history and may also see on your chart or hear the words *gravida* (grav'-uh-duh) and *para*. A *gravida* is a pregnant woman; you are a *primigravida* if you are now pregnant for the first time; a *multigravida* has been pregnant before (even if the pregnancy resulted in a spontaneous or deliberate abortion). *Para* refers to deliveries past the twentieth week of pregnancy—for example, a *primipara* is a woman who has delivered, by that definition, once.

The doctor will also give you an internal pelvic examination at this time.

Objective signs of pregnancy

During the pelvic, the examiner will be looking for internal signs of pregnancy to confirm your suspicion and the pregnancy test's accuracy. These signs, like the urine and blood tests, are called objective signs, although none is by itself a certain indication of pregnancy. They include:

1. *Goodell's sign.* After fertilization occurs, the vagina and cervix begin retaining fluid and softening. About six weeks after conception or two months after your last period (earlier in multigravidas), the change is discernible. Normally, the cervix feels hard, like the tip of a nose. During pregnancy, the cervix will feel soft, like lips.

2. *Hegar's sign.* With one hand on your abdomen and two fingers behind the cervix, the examiner can detect softening in the uterus at about the sixth week of gestation.

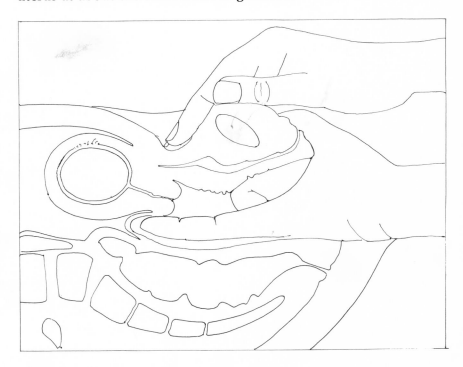

Fig. 2. Internal Examination for Pregnancy

3. *Chadwick's sign.* About eight weeks after conception, the vagina, vulva, and cervix appear bluish or dusky violet because of congestion and dilation of the veins.

The physician may detect other changes: enlargement of the uterus, changes in its shape from pearlike to globular, uterine bulges and soft spots where the embryo has implanted. In addition, if the examiner places fingers across the vagina, s/he may feel pronounced throbbing of the blood vessels. An examiner may also look for the "mask of pregnancy" and darkening of skin around the nipples.

By the time you've had a positive pregnancy test and begun prenatal care, a remarkable series of changes have already occurred within your body. Besides yourself, another being within you is undergoing an almost stupefying transformation from an infinitesimal single cell to a billion-celled human about twenty inches long and weighing approximately seven pounds.

Fetal development

Two weeks after fertilization   For about two weeks after ovulation, fertilized egg known as *ovum;* ovum moves down through Fallopian tube to uterus, where it implants.

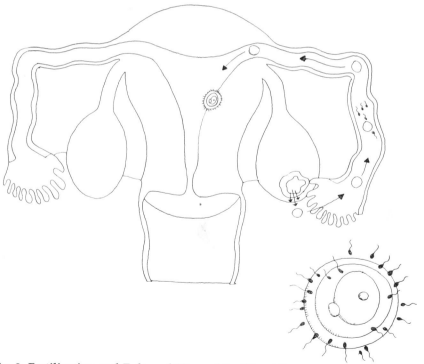

Fig. 3. Fertilization and Enlarged View of Fertilized Egg

Third week
after fertilization
Ovum now known as *embryo;* has cylindrical body with no human characteristics; rudimentary tubular heart begins to beat; lung and liver buds present; nervous system starts to develop; rudimentary eyes, spinal cord, and brain present.

Fourth week
after fertilization
Embryo is about one-fourth inch long at end of week; body curved so head and rudimentary tail almost meet; rudimentary nose and mouth present; prominent heart; arm and leg buds; digestive system forming; stalk that becomes umbilical cord present.

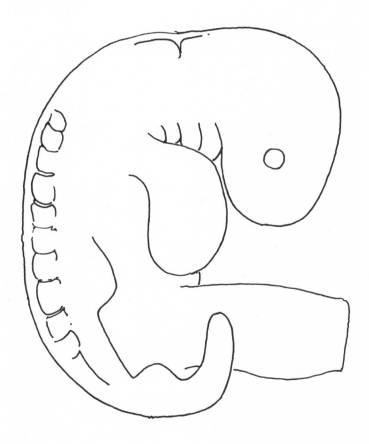

Fig. 4. Embryo at about Fourth Week after Fertilization

Sixth week after fertilization	Embryo is about seven-eighths of an inch long at end of week; large head in relation to trunk; face developing; external ears present; distinct nose; fingers and toes.
At the end of the second month of pregnancy	Embryo now known as *fetus;* begins to look distinctly human; about one and one-eighth of an inch long; head almost half fetus's size, eyes show pigmentation and begin shift from sides to front of head; eyelids fused; limbs begin rapid growth; hands and feet lose webbed look; heart chambers forming; lungs enlarge; digestive and circulatory systems growing; bones developing; gonads are differentiated; heartbeat pattern similar to an adult's.
At the end of the third month of pregnancy	Fetus is about three inches long; weighs one ounce; able to kick, make fists, suck thumb, curl toes, move head, squint; sometimes swallows amniotic fluid, then urinates back into amniotic fluid; external ears complete; hair follicles, teeth, bones, and muscles rapidly developing; skin thickens; limbs completely formed; nails on fingers and toes; vagina, uterus start to form; penis is distinct; bladder and kidneys develop; all major bodily systems exist, but not all are functioning.
At the end of the fourth month of pregnancy	Fetus is six to seven inches long; weighs about four ounces; transparent, reddish, and wrinkled skin; strong heartbeat; sex clearly distinguishable; eyes, ears, nose, and mouth approximate "normal" appearance; bony skeleton developing.
At the end of the fifth month of pregnancy	Fetus is about ten inches long; weighs one-half to one pound; some hair may be present on head; eyebrows and eyelashes appear; fine, downy hair called lanugo (luh-noo'-go) covers body; skin still red but less transparent; sweat glands forming; nipples develop; fetal organs well developed; lungs, skin, and digestive system not prepared to function outside womb.
At the end of the sixth month of pregnancy	Fetus is eleven to fourteen inches long; eyelids separated; eyes structurally complete; skin still wrinkled, but fat starts to be deposited beneath it; creamy, cheeselike coating, vernix caseosa (vur'-niks ka-see-o'-sah), covers skin; bone development advanced; ligaments, rings, and joints of spine begin to form.

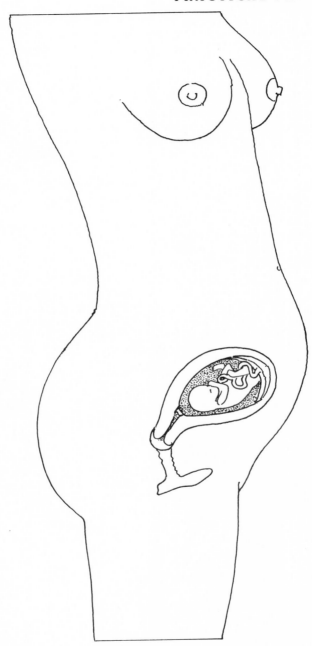

Fig. 5. The Third Month of Pregnancy

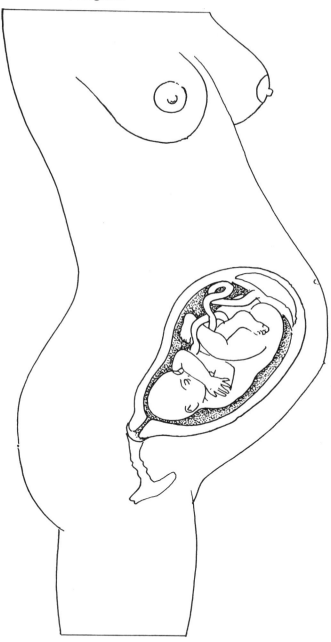

Fig. 6. The Sixth Month of Pregnancy

At the end of the seventh month of pregnancy

Fetus is fourteen to sixteen inches long; weighs two to three pounds; skin still red and wrinkled; lanugo begins to recede; brain well developed and integrating with nervous system; usually male's testes descend from abdomen into scrotal sac.

At the end of the eighth month of pregnancy

Fetus is sixteen to eighteen inches long; weighs four to five pounds; fat deposited under skin starts to smooth wrinkles; skin less red.

At the end of the ninth month of pregnancy

Fetus is about twenty inches long; weighs six to eight pounds; skin smooth and usually still coated with vernix; lanugo has mostly disappeared; maternal antibodies pass to fetus, offering temporary immunity to some diseases; nails go beyond tips of fingers and toes; head usually has covering of hair; nose and ear cartilage well developed; bones of head well developed.

Maternal development

First trimester

Uterus itself weighs about two ounces before pregnancy begins; typical uterine pear shape for first few weeks of pregnancy, then organ becomes more globular; by end of third month, shape is spherical. Fundus, or top of uterus, is in pelvis; uterine walls thin as pregnancy advances. Cessation of ovulation and menstruation, though some women bleed during first trimester at time of period. Woman may experience nausea, constipation, water retention. Increase in appetite; weight gain begins. Breasts often swell and throb; may increase in size; breast veins become more pronounced; nipples and areola may enlarge and darken. Cervix softens and becomes bluish; vulva and vagina become bluish, and vagina enlarges and secretes more. Ovaries and Fallopian tubes begin to change their positions. Woman may urinate more as growing uterus begins to press on bladder. Liver and kidneys seem to be undergoing changes. Increased oxygen consumption begins. Gradual elevation of diaphragm and flaring of ribs. Most cardiovascular changes occur now; by the end of the first trimester, cardiac output increases 25 to 50 percent; walls of blood vessels have a looser texture; increase in total plasma volume begins. Gums may swell, soften, and bleed more fre-

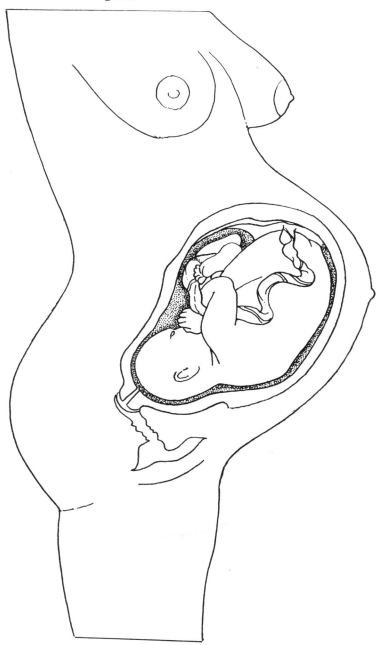

Fig. 7. The Ninth Month of Pregnancy

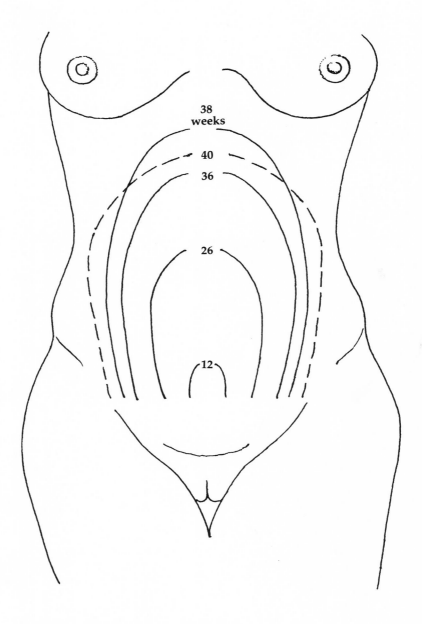

Fig. 8. Height of the Fundus During Pregnancy

quently. Skin may start to itch due to bile salt retention. Joints between pelvic bones widen. Body is storing protein, fat, minerals; increased need for iron. Endocrine glands producing a variety of hormones. Woman may start to experience mild emotional disturbances, such as depression or anxiety, or may feel euphoric.

Second trimester Uterus becomes increasingly distended and begins to displace other internal organs, such as stomach and intestines. Uterus assumes oval shape that remains until end of pregnancy; by end of fifth month, fundus of uterus reaches umbilicus. Woman experiences painless uterine contractions (Braxton-Hicks contractions). Woman's waist begins to disappear. Rapid increase in plasma volume. Cardiac output increases another 10 percent by end of second trimester; heart is shifting position and enlarging slightly. "Mask of pregnancy" may appear on face because of darkening skin pigment; skin on breasts, thighs, and abdomen stretches, and red or pink streaks may appear there. Vertical line from navel to pubic region darkens. Relaxation of smooth muscle in gastrointestinal tract may increase heartburn and cause bowels to move less efficiently. Increased perspiration and salivation. Colostrum may emerge from nipples. Fetal movements distinctly felt by woman. Second trimester often is a period of increased energy and euphoria for woman.

Third trimester Uterus weighs about two pounds at term. By ninth month, fundus of uterus is under woman's ribs. Two to four weeks before delivery (earlier in primigravida than multigravida), "lightening" occurs: uterus moves downward and out as fetal head engages in pelvis. More pressure may be exerted on bladder and rectum with lightening, but breathing should be easier. Large uterus changes body's center of gravity: walking may become more difficult and lower back pain may increase. Slight increase in plasma volume. Bladder and other internal organs increasingly displaced toward end of pregnancy. During the third trimester, many women experience sense of fatigue and depression that lasts until birth.

CHAPTER TWO
Choosing an Obstetrician/ Birth Attendant

One of the most important choices you make when you're pregnant is that of a birth attendant—the person who will monitor you throughout pregnancy and help you deliver your baby. The decision is important because it can make the difference between an informed, healthy pregnancy and one experienced in confused isolation; between a confident, comfortable labor and one over which you have little control; between a memorable delivery and one you'd rather forget; and between a healthy baby and one in distress.

Physician or midwife?

The first choice you may make involves the training of your birth attendant. Outside the United States, 80 percent of babies are delivered by midwives, but here the physician is dominant, delivering some 95 percent of infants. Yet the obstetrician is not your only alternative. Lay midwives still practice in this country. In some states they are legal. In other states they are not. A new breed of obstetric caretaker, the nurse-midwife, is finding widespread acceptance. Among physicians, you may choose an obstetrician, a family-practice specialist, or a general practitioner.

Your choice of caretaker will rest on certain facts and feelings. If you have a regular obstetrician-gynecologist, you may, through habit or conviction, remain with her/him during your pregnancy. Women should keep in mind, however, that caring for the pregnant patient is a good deal different from taking a Pap smear. A woman who stays with her gynecologist through her pregnancy should ask the same questions she would of a new doctor, and be sure that her feelings and wishes about birth will be respected.

Man or woman?

Because 92 percent of all obstetricians are men, there are limited options available to those of us who want to be attended by a woman. That's unfortunate because it's a natural impulse: first, because birth is uniquely woman's work; and second, because many of us simply feel more comfortable with another woman during so personal an experience. In fact, up until a hundred years ago, when male doctors started gaining a monopoly over childbirth, most American women went through labor and delivery with a female birth attendant. Many times, the quality of support and encouragement offered by a midwife is invaluable. It's sometimes hard to establish that kind of relationship with a male physician, since many expectant mothers are uncomfortable with the role they feel they must play (charming, respectful, cute). You will have to look hard to find one of the 8 percent of obstetricians who are women, one of the eighteen hundred certified nurse-midwives, or one of the licensed or unlicensed lay midwives scattered throughout the country.

Home or hospital?

Another factor determining the choice of your birth attendant is where you plan to deliver. If a particular hospital appeals to you because of its policies (for example, sibling visitation, rooming-in, encouragement of breast-feeding), you will have to select a physician with privileges at that hospital. In some hospitals, only board-certified *obstetricians* have staff privileges; in others, specialists in family practice and general practitioners may also deliver babies and perform necessary surgical and medical procedures related to delivery. If the hospital has a nurse-midwife program (few do, however), you will have that option. Lay midwives cannot practice in hospitals.

If you choose birth at home, you are restricted by law and by the availability of help. To find out how local laws may affect having a baby at home, your best bet is to speak with home-birth attendants in your area. In addition, the National Association of Parents and Professionals for Safe Alternatives in Childbirth (NAPSAC), P.O. Box 267, Marble Hill, MO 63764, keeps abreast of the latest legal developments affecting home birth. In most communities there are few or no doctors willing to attend a home birth. It's fair to say that most doubt its safety; in some cases, physicians may lose hospital privileges or malpractice insurance if they do de-

liveries at home. Parents committed to this option often face a di-
lemma. They may encounter a long search through licit or illicit
channels to find an experienced midwife (perhaps finding, ultimately, only inexperienced help), or they may elect, for want of alternatives, to deliver the baby themselves.

Your expectations

Later in this chapter, we will discuss the different qualifications and kinds of training of the various obstetric personnel. We
will list some of the questions you may want to ask before you en-
gage an individual to guide you through pregnancy and attend
your baby's birth. First, however, it may help to organize your
thoughts about what you expect from a physician, certified nurse-
midwife, or lay midwife.

• *Expertise.* Birth is a normal physiological process, although
we Americans sometimes seem to forget that. Our vast array of fetal monitors, IVs, anesthetics, drugs, forceps, and surgical procedures obscures the fact that 90 percent of all births need only be
monitored, not managed. In the other 10 percent, however, problems arise, whether during pregnancy, birth, or postpartum, and
then it is crucial to have an attendant who not only can recognize
complications immediately but can also marshal the technological
tools that may be lifesaving for you or your baby.

A woman giving birth at home, aided by an unlicensed attendant with little experience, must seriously consider the possibility
of being in that 10 percent problem group. She should be sure not
only that her attendant can *recognize* complications as early as possible, but also that the attendant has access to medication, hospitals,
and other professionals who can handle life-threatening complications.

A woman delivering in a hospital who seeks a birth with minimal technological intervention has the opposite problem. In advance, she should be satisfied that if she is in the 90 percent normal
group, her wishes regarding such things as anesthesia, fetal monitoring, or immediate bonding with the baby will be respected. It is
very difficult to argue about such procedures in the middle of labor.

• *Compatibility.* You will have many questions and, possibly, a
need for support and assurance. It is important to consider beforehand whether you expect these needs to be met by your physician

or midwife. If you do, you may be happier with an individual who can give freely of her/his time. Furthermore, women who know how they would like to structure their births, and who would like certain procedures (or would like those procedures eliminated), should not choose an attendant who will make them feel hesitant or upset about asking questions. It is terribly frustrating if the individual you depend on considers you, at best, bothersome and misguided, or, at worst, neurotic!

Some couples, especially those who already have children, have a very clear idea of the kind of birth they want. They have analyzed their previous experiences or studied the options. They come to a physician with a "shopping list" and are hopeful their wishes will be respected. They need an attendant who believes that the birthing couple's choices are most important, an individual who sees the need for adequate discussion when a request cannot be honored.

Moreover, couples who have not thought out their birth plans precisely deserve explanations of procedures, opportunities to make decisions, and recommendations about childbirth-education groups and literature.

Now, a look at those who help us deliver.

Physicians

A practicing physician has ordinarily completed four years of medical school. About 95 percent have completed an additional year of internship or residency training; most will have completed two or more years. S/he is licensed by the state in which s/he practices. Any physician (or nonphysician, depending on state law) can deliver babies. It is mostly obstetricians, family-practice specialists, and general practitioners who do so.

• *General practitioner.* The general practitioner may have no specialty training. Usually, s/he has completed four years of medical school and at least one year of graduate training, and is licensed by the state in which s/he practices. Because s/he lacks formal training in obstetrics, the general practitioner often does not have obstetrics privileges in major teaching hospitals, or is barred in some hospitals from performing such procedures as surgery or forceps delivery. S/he probably has privileges at a community hospital.

• *Family physician.* The family physician is a relatively new type of specialist. S/he has three years of graduate training in family medicine, which includes obstetrics, and may emphasize a particular area of family medicine, practicing with others who specialize in complementary fields. To be certified by the American Board of Family Practice, the individual generally will have completed four years of medical school and at least three years of graduate training, and have passed the board's specialty examination.

• *Obstetrician-gynecologist.* The obstetrician-gynecologist is a physician who specializes in the treatment of conditions related to the female reproductive organs. Although any physician may call her/himself a "specialist" in obstetrics, certification by the American Board of Obstetrics and Gynecology indicates intensive graduate training and successful completion of the board's oral and written examinations.

Board certification may be a way to judge medical competence, but it indicates nothing about personal attributes, or what used to be called a "bedside manner." And of course there are, no doubt, excellent obstetricians who have just never gotten around to fulfilling board requirements. Always shop carefully when choosing a physician. (Sometimes an obstetrician will have the initials F.A.C.O.G. after her/his name. This means that the individual is a fellow of the American College of Obstetricians and Gynecologists, a voluntary association. To be a fellow, the obstetrician must have completed graduate training, be board-certified, and have practiced for at least five years.)

How to find a doctor

Start your search for a physician by questioning friends about theirs or, if necessary, by looking in the Yellow Pages or by calling local hospitals for recommendations. Ask friends how they felt about pre- and postnatal care and how deliveries were handled. If you're looking for a specialist, ask your family doctor for some suggestions. When you have some names, you may want to check their qualifications and licensing with your state's physicians' licensing authority. Alternatively, call the county medical association or the hospital where the physician has staff privileges to ask about her/his education, residency training, and experience. (Don't waste valuable time and goodwill discussing these questions with the physician's office personnel or the physician her/himself. Do your own legwork.)

Next, divide questions you have into those that you can ask office personnel and those that you must ask the doctor at a scheduled appointment. Call the physician's office and ask the nurse when you may call back with some questions about the practice. You are more likely to get time and attention this way than you would in a rushed, midday conversation.

Questions to ask office personnel

1. *How much do the physician's services cost and what does the fee include?*

Obstetric fees are usually a package: one price covers prenatal care, delivery, and postnatal checkup. Depending on your location, fees may run as low as $350 or as high as $2,000 and more. Laboratory tests (blood, urine, and others) will be extra but are generally standard in price. A cesarean section, should it be necessary, will also increase your bill—ask by how much. Finally, if it is important that you know, find out the fee billing schedule—by what date the total fee must be paid.

Note that hospital costs are separate from physician's fees. Once you know the physician's hospital affiliation, you can call the business office to find out the cost of an average, uncomplicated delivery and add that to the physician's fee to determine your total estimated birth cost.

2. *What is the physician's attitude toward prepared childbirth?*

If the nurse hesitates, laughs, or says, "Maybe you should speak to the doctor," this may not be the place for you if you want a prepared birth. The nurse most probably is reflecting the doctor's attitude. On the other hand, an enthusiastic "Yes!" may not be too informative because nowadays the phrase "prepared childbirth" can mean just about anything. While once it may have meant minimum intervention, today some physicians and mothers will discuss a "prepared childbirth" that includes spinal anesthesia, internal fetal monitoring, forceps, and episiotomy. All of these are procedures that many of the pioneers of prepared childbirth rejected for the majority of cases.

3. *How many partners are in the practice?*

Often, physicians practice together and take turns being "on call" for deliveries. If yours is not on duty the day you go into labor, you may be attended by a doctor you've never met or barely know. Obviously, a couple patronizing a two-partner practice is more likely to know the birth attendant than a couple enrolled in a much larger practice or a clinic. If a large practice lacks intimacy, it has the advantage of pooled skills and specialties. It also has the advantage of convenience, since a variety of laboratory and birth-monitoring equipment may be right on the premises. Should you need lab work or, for example, ultrasound, this can be done by your physician in the office, not at a distant hospital. (Of course, a vast array of equipment may increase costs unnecessarily. Some practitioners may be inclined to use it simply because it's there or because it must be paid for.)

4. *Which hospital is the physician affiliated with?*

In some ways, this may be the most important question you ask. Your best intentions (and your physician's!) about breast-feeding, rooming-in, or partner participation in the birth can be crushed by hospital regulations or traditions.

5. *How often will I see the physician?*

There is much variation among physicians in the number of regular visits they plan for their patients. Some want you in as soon as you miss a period; some ask you to wait two months. Some see you biweekly at first; others, monthly. And while most physicians see patients weekly during the last month, others begin the weekly schedule earlier, or not at all. The average, uncomplicated pregnancy will probably involve twelve to fourteen visits.

6. *How long will I have to wait at each visit?*

If you are talking to a particularly genial and frank employee, you might ask how long you can expect to be in the waiting room for each visit. This estimate may not prove accurate for each appointment but might help you somewhat in planning your workday, hiring a baby-sitter, and so on.

Questions for the doctor

If everything checks out favorably, make an appointment for a consultation. Explain that you'd like to speak with the physician and ask some questions. Most likely, there will be a fee. If you can't get to all the following questions, ask only the ones most important to *you*.

1. *How do you feel about my partner's participation in prenatal care, labor, and delivery?*

If the physician seems uncomfortable with this concept, yet it is important to you to have loving support during pregnancy and birth, this physician is not for you (s/he may not provide the comfort you need if your partner isn't there). And your partner's participation means just that: accompanying you to office exams if you wish; staying with you throughout labor and delivery; being able to hold the baby soon after delivery; sitting with you in the recovery room. Some physicians ask husbands or partners to leave during vaginal exams in labor or in their offices. There really is no reason for this exclusion, and during labor it is particularly valuable to have someone helping you breathe and relax if internals are uncomfortable.

Remember that despite the recent upsurge in family-centered maternity care, some hospitals still do not permit husbands or partners to accompany women during labor and delivery. If you like the physician and can live with the hospital's limits, stay with the practice (ask, though, what s/he is doing to liberalize hospital rules). You can always hope there will be some sympathetic nurses on duty when you're in labor.

Finally, if you wish to have someone other than your partner, or in addition to your partner, with you during labor and/or delivery, then find out *now* about the hospital's or physician's rules.

2. *Do you encourage parents to take childbirth-education classes?*

Press on if the answer is yes, for that may imply that the physician is comfortable with a woman in control of labor and that s/he favors minimal use of medication during the birth experience.

3. *How do you feel about breast-feeding? Bottle-feeding?*

The doctor's views should be compatible with yours.

4. *Do you routinely perform an episiotomy?*

An episiotomy (i-piz-ee-aht'-uh-mee) is an incision made in the perineum (per-uh-nee'-um) (the pelvic floor) that widens the vaginal opening. After delivery, the incision is sutured. Because the surgically enlarged perineum doesn't have to stretch so far, delivery is accomplished more quickly. Also, some physicians believe that without an episiotomy the constant pounding of the baby's head against the perineum may be harmful, particularly if this stage of labor is lengthy. Finally, some physicians say an incision is necessary to avoid a jagged tear. Episiotomies in this country are routine, but not so in the rest of the world. The stitches may be uncomfortable during the postnatal period; you may find it hard to walk or sit at first. Sometimes the pain—actual or remembered—inhibits you from having sex. Physicians and midwives who do not perform episiotomies say the procedure is rarely necessary when a woman has good control over her perineal muscles, when the attendant supports the perineum and uses warm cloths and massage to help it soften, or when birth is not rushed and tissues are allowed to stretch gradually.

5. *How do you feel about maternal-infant bonding immediately after delivery?*

Ever since two researchers, Dr. Marshall Klaus and Dr. John Kennell, wrote about the importance of interaction between mother and baby immediately after birth, professionals have been seeking ways to encourage this kind of bonding. If early bonding is important to you, make sure you are allowed to do some of the following: hold your baby immediately after birth; nurse on the delivery table or in the recovery room; have the father hold the infant; delay silver-nitrate drops (they are irritating and may temporarily impair the baby's vision); have the baby with you in the recovery room or at your bedside in your own hospital room.

6. *Can you arrange the birth setting so that it is similar to the environment Dr. Frederick Leboyer suggests?*

Birth Without Violence, by Dr. Leboyer, caused quite a stir a few years back by suggesting babies be delivered in tranquil settings: with the delivery room dimly lighted, the baby being given a quiet, warm bath and placed on the mother's abdomen. If these conditions appeal to you, perhaps your physician can duplicate or at least modify your birth in accordance with Dr. Leboyer's suggestions.

7. *What prepping procedures are routine? Can any be modified?*

Usually, when admitted to a hospital, a woman in labor is given an enema and has at least some pubic hair shaved. There is much debate about whether either of these procedures is necessary. (Of course, neither is usually painful, but they are annoyances.) If the thought of prepping disturbs you, discuss it with the doctor. In addition, attaching an IV is a routine procedure. The IV may drip sugar-water solution for energy, or it may be hooked up "just in case" you need an anesthetic or other medication administered intravenously. But an IV can impede mobility, especially when you have to go to the bathroom. Ask if you can do without it.

8. *What anesthetics and analgesics do you routinely instruct the hospital staff to dispense?*

Whether you want to go through labor with no medication, or whether you feel comfortable about receiving pain relievers, it's important to know in advance which drugs your physician will administer. Find out what s/he offers during labor and delivery—including the side effects, the benefits, the effects on the baby and on the labor and delivery. In addition, a physician who employs the same procedure for every birth should be avoided. Be certain her/his plans are individualized.

Often, physicians will actually give their patients a choice of anesthetics or analgesics, so you should know *in advance* the kinds of drugs you may be offered. If you don't think about this until labor begins, you can hardly expect to make an informed decision.

9. *What percentage of your patients have cesarean births?*

The incidence of cesarean birth has risen dramatically in recent years. In some hospitals, an incredible 40 percent of all births are abdominal. While no one can say what an optimum percentage would be for every practice (the percentage depends on the type of patients), critics wonder whether all the surgery done today is justified. In addition, a study done in Rhode Island and published in the *New England Journal of Medicine* found a higher mortality rate for mothers delivering abdominally than for those delivering vaginally. What cesarean percentage is acceptable? Some groups claim 10 percent—for an obstetrician. The case load of a general practitioner who cannot perform this surgery her/himself may reflect a lower percentage; a practice that serves a high-risk population may reflect a greater percentage of cesarean births.

10. *How long must I stay in the hospital?*

To some women with no insurance or with little children at home, the prospect of even a three-day hospital stay is upsetting. Some physicians are cutting hospital stays to twenty-four hours if there's good reason and mother and baby are doing well.

11. *Do you impose any dietary or weight-gain restrictions on your patients?*

Increasing evidence indicates that pregnancy is not the time to diet, limit weight gain, limit salt intake, or take appetite suppressants or diuretics to control weight. Weight gains of thirty pounds or more may be perfectly acceptable and beneficial to your baby. Seriously question a physician who has rigid notions about dieting.

If you are a vegetarian, you will also want to know if your physician feels comfortable and knowledgeable about your care. In certain cases, vegetarian women will need different kinds of vitamin supplements.

12. *Can I be sure my wishes concerning birth will be complied with by the hospital and by whoever attends my birth?*

Your physician should let you know that if your requests are not part of her/his standing orders, they will be noted on your chart, and that the chart will accompany you in the hospital.

If when the visit draws to a close you are not sure about committing yourself, don't. Take time, later, to assess the answers you've received. Also, consider the physician's:

• **Demeanor.** Was s/he responsive and interested in your questions, or condescending and bored? Were you rushed, or listened to carefully? Did you feel you were treated as an adult, or did you feel patronized?

• *Age.* Some women want to be sure their obstetricians will be around to deliver all their babies and to take care of their gynecological needs for the long run; they prefer younger physicians. Other women are more comfortable with older doctors who have had more extensive experience.

• *Attitude on equality.* Many women object to calling the physician Dr. So-and-So, while being addressed by their first name. It's a valid point but probably hopelessly irremediable.

Other issues will arise during your pregnancy that cannot be explored in the initial interview. Does your physician remember your name? Give you an opportunity to dress and collect yourself before you discuss your questions? Rush out of the examining room? Avoid conversation? Encourage questions? Answer them in detail? Seem to be interested in you as an individual rather than as a reproductive organ?

If your physician is a general practitioner or family specialist, some other points are worth considering. If you need a cesarean, who will perform it? (In some hospitals, this kind of surgery cannot be done by nonspecialists.) In addition, consider whether your physician will be caring for your baby after birth. If so, ask friends about her/his experience and qualities as a pediatrician. *You* might not mind a brusque manner, but a toddler may not react favorably. Office location is a factor, too. You are more apt to need propinquity when dealing with your child's physician than when dealing with an obstetrician.

Rarely will you find a physician who can meet your needs completely; after all, physicians are human and have their own preferences and standards. Ultimately, every woman must judge for herself which of her needs are paramount and on which points she's willing to compromise.

Certified nurse-midwife

As of mid-1979, there were only eighteen hundred certified nurse-midwives in the United States. In 1976—the last year for which statistics are available—they delivered only about 1 percent of our newborns, but already they have made an impact on the way we look at birth. More and more, we are beginning to see most births as normal physiological occurrences that require only watchful waiting and emotional support by a skilled attendant. We are beginning to see that our highly trained physicians may have skills more matched to those few births that may be complicated or hazardous.

It is for the normal birth that the CNM is ideally trained. The philosophy of the American College of Nurse-Midwives (ACNM) states, in part: "Every childbearing family has a right to a safe, satisfying maternity experience with respect for human dignity and worth; for variety in cultural forms; and for the parents' right to self-determination."

To be certified, the CNM must be a registered nurse, must have completed a one- or two-year educational program at a school recognized by the ACNM, and must have passed a certification examination administered by the college. Some nurse-midwives also complete internships. The American College of Obstetricians and Gynecologists (ACOG) has recognized this specialty since 1971. In a joint statement on maternity care with the American College of Nurse-Midwives, the ACOG said: " . . . qualified nurse-midwives may assume responsibility for the complete care and management of uncomplicated maternity patients." According to the report, *Nurse-Midwifery in the United States 1976–77,* "As of December, 1977, the practice of nurse-midwifery, including management of labor and delivery, was recognized in the laws of all states except Michigan, Missouri and Wisconsin."

The CNM works under the ultimate direction of a physician, with whom she may consult or to whom she refers cases with complications. But depending on the practice or the hospital with which she is affiliated, her responsibilities vary. Many CNMs deliver babies; some give only prenatal care; some can handle multiple births; a fraction even do home births. Some of the different duties of the nurse-midwife, as compiled by the ACNM, include: diagnosing pregnancy and giving prenatal physical examinations; managing some complications; staying with patients during labor; applying fetal monitors; performing home deliveries, episiotomies, forceps deliveries, newborn resuscitation, circumcision, and well-baby care.

Because they are so few, nurse-midwives are hard to find. Some are with public health agencies or hospitals; others practice privately (with medical backup), or in association with physicians. Many can be found in maternity centers.

Why choose a certified nurse-midwife? Barbara Brennan, a CNM, explains in her book *The Complete Book of Midwifery:* "Profes-

sional midwives look at pregnancy and childbirth as a normal process, something a woman's body is designed to do and can do by
itself 9 times out of 10—by giving the woman little more than reas-
surance, encouragement, guidance, and a pair of helping hands."
Any woman who has had a nurse-midwife sit patiently and en-
couragingly with her for hours of labor knows the truth of this.

Which is not to say that an obstetrician could not give this
kind of care—some do. But the fact is that most physicians are men
and perhaps not so attuned as another woman would be to a laboring woman's needs and feelings. Having a highly technical education, some obstetricians find it hard to monitor a normal, eighteen-
hour labor patiently, and only a small number would sit with a laboring woman for any length of time. Brennan also points out that
specialists may be overtrained for the normal birth, while the normal birth is the nurse-midwife's exclusive concern.

Other reasons to seek out a nurse-midwife? The fee is lower,
and often, because she has few gynecologic patients and few emergencies, the nurse-midwife has more time to devote to her pregnant patients. Many CNMs are so adamant about working *with*
women during labor that they insist patients take prepared-childbirth classes. And some are so dedicated to fulfilling couples' wishes that they will deliver at home.

Opting for a nurse-midwife, however, does not guarantee a
particular kind of birth. You should not hesitate to ask the CNM
the same questions you would ask a physician about your care.
You should determine whether the nurse-midwife is certified, and
find out about her background, training, education, and experience. And then, add the following:

1. *If complications arise during my pregnancy, to which physician will I
be referred? Will I have a choice of physicians? Will I meet them at some point
during my pregnancy?*

2. *If a last-minute emergency arises, requiring a cesarean, who will perform it? Will you be with me during surgery?*

3. *Do you administer postnatal care? Later gynecologic care? Well-baby
examinations?*

4. *Who will be present at my birth (doctors, other nurse-midwives, obstetrics nurses)?*

5. (For those delivering in maternity centers—institutions that
care only for maternity patients—rather than hospitals:) *What is the
backup hospital if an emergency arises? How far away is it? Under what conditions are patients transferred there? Will you accompany me?*

It is important to point out that nurse-midwives cannot accept
each woman who wishes to be a patient, because some women

need the kind of care only an obstetrics specialist can provide. For example, depending on which complications they handle, a CNM may refer to physicians women who:

- have a history of kidney or heart disease, hypertension, diabetes, epilepsy
- have had a previous cesarean birth
- have frequently aborted
- have Rh problems

During pregnancy, a woman may have to transfer to a physician's care if:

- she has preeclampsia
- the baby is in an abnormal position
- there is a multiple pregnancy
- there is abnormal uterine bleeding
- cephalopelvic disproportion is suspected (the baby may be too large to fit through the mother's bony pelvis)
- it is suspected that the baby is abnormal

A physician may be called into labor and delivery if:

- labor does not begin within twelve to twenty-four hours after membranes have ruptured
- fetal heart tones are abnormal
- labor does not progress
- there is abnormal bleeding
- the umbilical cord has prolapsed (slipped out before the baby)

For more information, contact the American College of Nurse-Midwives, 1012 Fourteenth Street, N.W., Suite 801, Washington, D.C. 20005.

Prenatal care

Good prenatal care, whether administered by a physician or a nurse-midwife, is essential for your health and that of your baby. Care should begin as early as possible—certainly by the end of the first trimester—yet it is shocking to realize that some 28 percent of all American women have received no prenatal care by that time.

What constitutes prenatal care? Let's take a look at an average pregnancy.

Generally, a pregnant woman will see her physician once a month during the first seven months, every two weeks until the ninth month, then weekly until birth. Some physicians and CNMs may schedule more frequent visits; a complicated case may *require* more visits—sometimes weekly from conception to birth.

The first visit

A medical record will be set up that includes a health and family history. In addition to your name, phone number, address, occupation, and health insurance arrangements, you will be asked about: (1) the current or suspected pregnancy; (2) previous pregnancies and abortions; (3) your menstrual history and any irregularities; (4) surgery and medications; (5) past disorders, infections, and diseases; (6) family members and their state of health. You should offer information about physical stress and any potentially toxic chemicals you may be exposed to at work or at home.

After your history, a physical examination will begin with your height, weight, and blood pressure measurements; and then, often, an external examination will be performed that includes the ears, nose, and throat, palpation of the thyroid, listening to the heart and lungs, and palpation of the breasts and abdomen. If you have a particular medical problem, you will be questioned carefully about it, and your answers may determine the nature of your physical examination. A specialist may be brought into your case.

Usually, an internal (pelvic) examination will also be performed at a first visit. Your physician or midwife may be: (1) actually confirming your pregnancy; (2) checking on the health of your reproductive organs; (3) determining the size and shape of your bony pelvis; and (4) determining the size of your uterus and the age of the fetus. Obtaining accurate information at this point may eliminate the need for expensive tests later on.

You will have blood drawn so that a complete blood count can be done, as well as tests for rubella, syphilis, blood type, and Rh status. A tuberculin test may be performed. You will have to void a urine specimen, and sometimes a Pap smear will be taken, too. Patients at risk may also be tested or questioned about genetic disorders such as sickle-cell anemia, or infectious diseases such as toxoplasmosis.

The final component of your initial visit is usually a discussion about nutrition; health habits; sex and physical activity during pregnancy; the schedule of office visits and outline of care; phone calls and emergencies; physiology; and general future plans for delivery. If you don't already know, ask about fees, books, and pamphlets. Also, you will be told about the danger signs: abnormal bleeding, abdominal pain, blurred vision, painful headache, severe vomiting, or pain on urination.

Don't rush this visit—physicians and midwives are well aware that the initial appointment is often lengthy. Although many questions about labor and delivery can be postponed for several months, issues you are seriously concerned about should be brought up now.

Subsequent visits

At every visit, your weight and blood pressure will be taken and your urine will be tested for protein and glucose. In some offices, patients are taught how to test urine themselves and to record the results. After the initial internal exam, the remainder of your examinations will probably be external *unless* you are experiencing bleeding, there is a question about fetal age, or you have a history of habitual abortion—in which case your cervix must be checked regularly for signs of dilatation.

During the external examination, the physician or midwife will be checking the height of the top of the uterus and the rate and location of the baby's heartbeat. The heartbeat first becomes discernible at about the third month of pregnancy; it can be heard by the mother, too, if the examiner uses a Doppler probe. (A Doppler probe is a small rectangular or flashlight-shaped device that uses ultrasonic waves to detect the fetal heartbeat. The probe is moved along the mother's abdomen until the heart tones are picked up.) You will also be checked for signs of puffiness and abnormalities. Because your questions and comments will direct the course of the examination, don't be hesitant about discussing what's on your mind. At some point, too, your caretaker should be recommending prepared-childbirth and baby-care classes. Although there are many classes you do not enter until your last trimester, it is important to sign up early.

During the middle part of pregnancy, depending on your health, you may have more laboratory tests—for hemoglobin or diabetes, for example. Women with kidney problems may have a urine culture every three months. And, of course, all the tests listed in Chapter 3 may be performed, too, at different stages.

The last month

Internal examinations should begin again. Physicians will be able to feel the baby abdominally and determine its size and posi-

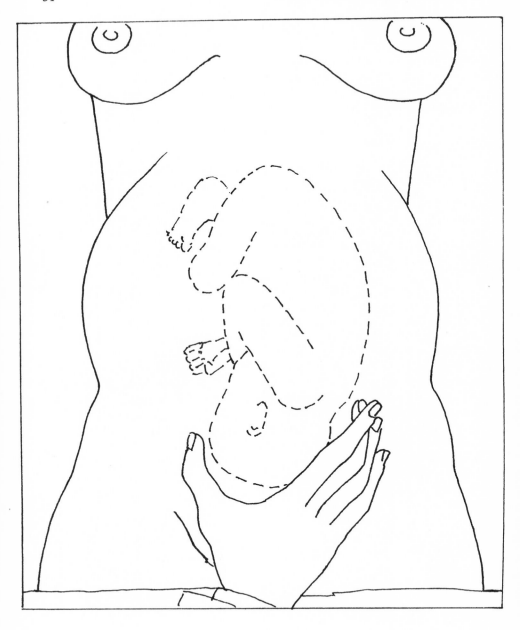

Fig. 9. External Examination of Fetal Size and Position

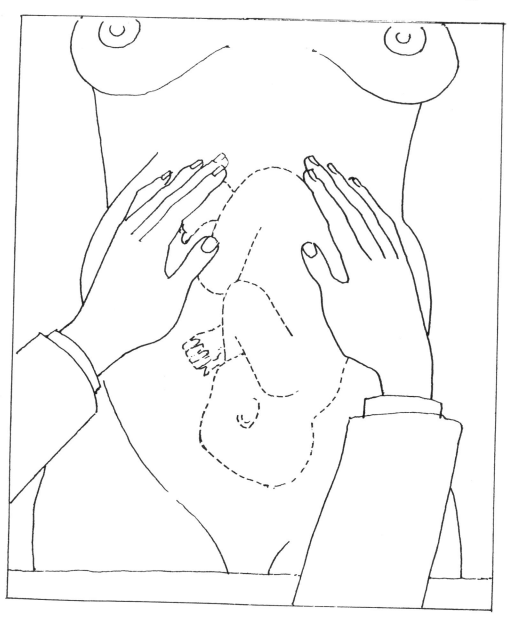

2099087

tion. Internal examinations will disclose descent of the baby's head, condition of the cervix, and imminence of birth, and will again serve to delineate the bony pelvis. Early in the last month you will be advised about how to recognize the onset of labor and at what point to notify the office.

During labor

If you are admitted in labor to a hospital, you will probably be checked first, if your own physician is not there, by the resident, attending physician, or nursing staff on duty. The purpose of this internal examination is to check the dilatation and effacement of your cervix. Your physician will be contacted with this information. S/he will probably arrive when you are in active labor. It helps to know that pelvic examinations are kept to a minimum—particularly if membranes have ruptured—to reduce the possibility of infection. During active labor, however, you may be examined internally as often as once an hour. Unfortunately, examinations during labor are often performed during contractions, when the dilatation of the cervix is greatest. This means the process may be painful.

After delivery, the birth attendant will check on you while you are in the recovery room.

During your stay in the hospital, your physician or nurse-midwife will visit you daily. In teaching institutions, the resident assigned to your case will also visit, but should authorize no treatment unless your physician approves. In all cases, the physician or nurse-midwife will be checking: (1) whether the uterus is well contracted; (2) the quantity of blood discharged; (3) the stitches and perineum if there is more than usual discomfort. Twenty-four hours before you leave the hospital, you should receive "going-home" instructions on postpartum activity, sex, exercise, and abnormal signs. If you deliver in a small hospital, with a small nursing staff and few or no postpartum classes, be sure to question your physicians (including pediatrician) on bottle-feeding, breast-feeding, bathing the baby, and all other postpartum or baby-care concerns you have.

Postpartum

Four to six weeks after delivery, or earlier if you have had a cesarean birth, you will have a postpartum checkup. It will include weight, blood pressure, examination of abdomen and breasts, urinalysis, and blood count. You will have a pelvic examination as well, to determine the size and health of your reproductive organs and to check stitches, if any. You should take this opportunity to discuss and obtain birth control devices.

CHAPTER THREE
Tests Before and During Pregnancy

In addition to tests for confirming pregnancy, women can undergo a variety of other tests, before and during pregnancy, to learn about their own health and that of the fetus.

Tests before pregnancy

From the moment she knows she's expecting, a woman imagines how her infant will look: if s/he will have brown hair or blond, blue eyes or green, will be husky or small. Every pregnant woman envisions a perfect child. We rarely admit even the possibility of problems—although according to The National Foundation–March of Dimes, birth defects affect approximately 250,000 American babies in some degree each year.

Past generations of pregnant women could only gamble that their children would be born healthy. Today, many disorders can be predicted and prevented, and the outcome of pregnancy is far less risky. Women needn't become pregnant before they know their chances of passing on birth defects. Information is available through prepregnancy testing and counseling about genetic make-up, health, and habits that will tell them about the health of their future children.

Genetic disorders

Some prepregnancy tests can identify genetic diseases a couple may carry and pass on to their children. Normally, every cell in the body carries forty-six chromosomes (in twenty-three pairs). The exceptions are the sex cells—egg and sperm—which contribute twenty-three chromosomes each to a new human being. Every chromosome carries thousands of genes, which in turn affect tens of thousands of human traits. Genes determine which characteristics are inherited from the parents, from height and hair color to the structure of internal organs and the manner in which the body performs its chemical processes. If either parent carries a defective gene or chromosome—and especially if both do—the children may be affected.

Generally, genetic disorders may be caused by: (1) abnormal structure, number, or arrangement of chromosomes; (2) dominant genes; (3) recessive genes; (4) genes located on the X chromosome; and (5) genes acting with other genes and environmental factors.

Chromosomal diseases

Most chromosomal diseases are not hereditary. A particular egg or sperm may be accidentally produced with the wrong number or makeup of chromosomes, but nature usually corrects such mistakes by aborting the deformed embryo or fetus. When the fetus survives to term, it may be afflicted with mental or physical problems ranging from mild to severe. A classic example of a serious chromosomal disorder is Down's syndrome (formerly called mongolism), in which the victim suffers mental retardation and physical maldevelopment. The most common form of Down's syndrome is known medically as trisomy 21. The vast majority of trisomy 21 cases are isolated accidents. Only about 3 percent are hereditary—the result of the parents being carriers of a chromosomal aberration known as a translocation abnormality.

You may suspect a hereditary chromosomal problem (and there are dozens besides Down's syndrome) if: (1) a relative has been identified as having or carrying a chromosomal disorder; (2) you have borne a child with a chromosomal disease; (3) you have suffered three or more consecutive miscarriages.

Before you get pregnant (or pregnant again), your doctor may recommend an analysis of tissue, usually your blood. From this blood sample, each of your chromosomes and its components are ordered and identified on a diagram called a karyotype (kar'-ee-uh-type), which allows specialists to see any abnormalities in chromosomal number or appearance.

Dominant genes

Every human being receives his or her genes equally from both parents. But some genes governing a specific human charac-

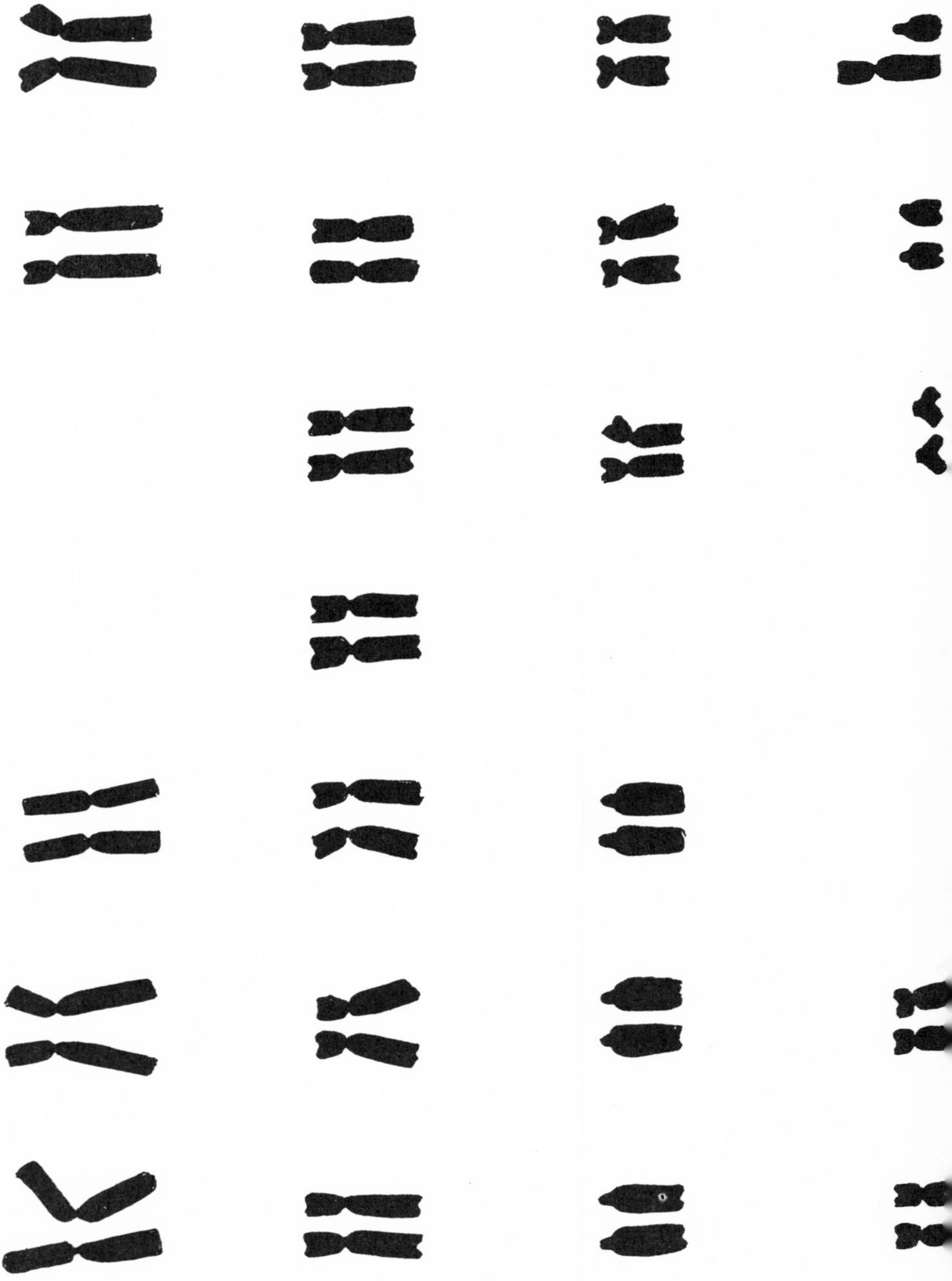

Fig. 10. Human Karyotype

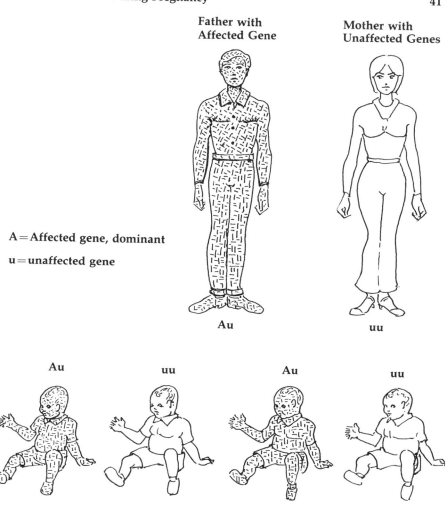

Fig. 11. Dominant Inheritance

teristic will dominate. For example, the gene for brown eyes dominates the gene for blue eyes. With harmless genes, dominance poses no problem. But when a gene that produces disease is dominant, only one parent need have the disease for each child conceived to have a 50 percent chance of inheriting it. Unlike chromosomal disorders, which are usually isolated accidents, many gene-produced diseases are hereditary, and the probability that your children will inherit them exists for each pregnancy.

Among the thousand or so identified dominant-gene disorders are Huntington's disease, a degenerative disease of the nervous system, which usually doesn't appear until the victim is about thirty years old; achondroplasia (a-kan-dro-pla'-zhuh), a type of dwarfism; and hypercholesterolemia (hi-puhr-kuh-les-tuh-ruh-lee'-mee-uh), in which high blood-cholesterol levels often lead to heart disease.

For these disorders, there are at present no tests *before* pregnancy to determine if your children will inherit the disease. And for a disease that appears later in life, such as Huntington's, afflicted individuals may not know they themselves have the disorder until they have already passed it on to their children. In such a case, the appearance of the disease in other members of your family should alert your doctor to the need for genetic studies and counseling.

Recessive genes

When a gene for a disease is recessive, rather than dominant, *both* parents must carry the gene before there is a chance their offspring will inherit the disease. Parents who are carriers of a recessive gene for a particular disease will not themselves be affected by the disorder. But if both carry it, the laws of heredity decree that for each pregnancy there is a 25 percent chance the child will have the disease, a 50 percent chance that the child will be a carrier, and a 25 percent chance that the child will neither have the disease nor be a carrier.

About a thousand known recessive-gene disorders exist, some of which seem to strike certain ethnic groups more frequently than others. Specific genetic diseases have been identified in a wide variety of ethnic groups, including South Africans, Eskimos, and Norwegians. Individuals can undergo simple tests to determine whether they carry genes for some of these diseases, and consider the outcome of a pregnancy before they begin having children.

Sickle-cell anemia

Sickle-cell anemia is one such recessive-gene disorder. In the United States, this disease strikes 1 out of every 400 to 600 black children. Persons of Mediterranean and Middle Eastern background may also carry the sickle-cell gene, which is thought to have evolved originally as a protection against malaria. Those who have one altered gene are said to carry the sickle-cell "trait." Earlier

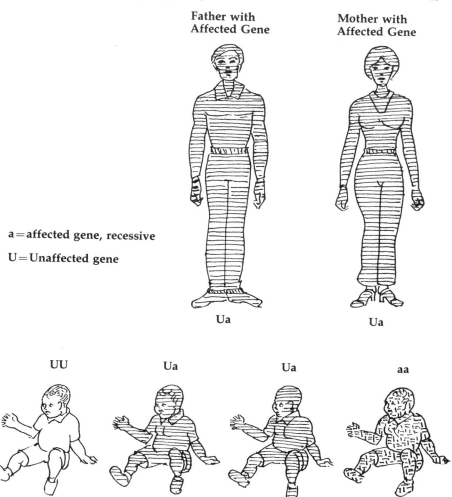

Father with
Affected Gene

Mother with
Affected Gene

a = affected gene, recessive

U = Unaffected gene

Ua

Ua

UU   Ua   Ua   aa

Fig. 12. Recessive Inheritance

medical opinions that even persons with the trait were somewhat physically and mentally afflicted have been refuted by recent studies.

In sickle-cell anemia, the altered genes cause red blood cells to take on an elongated, rather than normal spheroidal, shape—thus making their passage through small blood vessels difficult. Symptoms of the disorder include fatigue, shortness of breath, pallor, loss of appetite, and pain in the extremities, back, and abdomen.

Retarded physical development, illness, and often death may follow. A simple blood test, done in a doctor's office, or frequently offered through a local board of health, can determine whether you carry the sickle-cell trait *before* you get pregnant. In addition, many physicians routinely test all pregnant black women for sickle-cell disease or trait at the first or second prenatal visit.

Thalassemia

Another genetic anemia is thalassemia (thal-uh-see'-mee-uh), or Cooley's anemia. Almost 250,000 Americans are carriers of the gene for Cooley's anemia, and thousands of children suffer a severe form of the disease. Most of these individuals are of Greek or Italian ancestry, although persons of Chinese, Indian, and African heritage may also carry the gene. The gene that carries Cooley's anemia prevents normal production of hemoglobin, the essential oxygen carrier in red blood cells. Poor appetite, listlessness, and worsening infections are the first signs of this life-shortening disorder. Then the spleen and liver enlarge, and bones tend to become brittle. Through blood tests, physicians can determine the presence of Cooley's anemia or the trait.

Tay-Sachs disease

The Tay-Sachs gene apparently developed first in Jewish villages in northeastern Poland, and most carriers are Jews who trace their ancestry to this region. Scientists have recently discovered an Eastern European group of Mennonites in Pennsylvania and a French-Canadian Roman Catholic group in Quebec who also have the gene.

The Tay-Sachs gene prevents the body from producing a necessary enzyme, hexosaminidase A, or Hex A. Without the enzyme, fatty substances accumulate in the cells, most seriously in the victim's brain cells. Eventually, these cells expand. The brain begins to function less effectively, mental retardation and deafness set in, and death usually occurs by the age of four.

There is as yet no cure for this disease. But Jewish couples of Eastern European heritage can have their Hex A levels determined with a simple blood test before beginning a pregnancy. This blood test should not be done on a pregnant woman because false results will be obtained. However, if there is a history of Tay-Sachs disease in the family of either parent, the male partner will be tested at the first or second prenatal visit. If he is negative, no further testing is done. If he is positive, amniocentesis (see page 52) will be considered.

Cystic fibrosis

For some other well-known recessive-gene diseases, there are at present no tests to determine the carrier status of parents-to-be. One of the most widespread of these diseases is cystic fibrosis, the gene for which is carried by an estimated ten million Americans. In cystic fibrosis, the function of certain glands—mainly the mucous glands—is impaired, leading eventually to recurrent lung infections and digestive problems. Specialists are presently working on a test to identify cystic fibrosis carriers before a pregnancy begins.

X-linked diseases

Some inheritable diseases are transmitted only through genes on the X chromosomes. Normally, we all receive one sex chromosome from each parent: a woman has two X chromosomes and a man one X and one Y chromosome. The father, then, is responsible for the sex of the child: if he passes on an X chromosome, the child will be female; if he transmits the Y, then the child will be male. Unfortunately, almost two hundred diseases have been found to be caused by genes on the X chromosome, which may be carried by an unaffected female parent. These disorders are termed X-linked diseases, since no genetic problems have been specifically linked to the Y chromosome.

If a woman is a carrier of any X-linked disease, she has one normal X chromosome and one altered X chromosome, but she herself does not suffer from the disease. Her daughters may receive her normal X chromosome and be free of the disease. Or they may receive her altered X and be carriers like their mother. In the latter case, the father's normal X chromosome in essence "neutralizes" the effects of the mother's altered X. The mother may also transmit her normal X chromosome to her sons. But if the mother transmits her altered X chromosome, and the father contributes a Y chromosome, the Y has no gene to counterbalance the altered X, and the son will suffer from the disease.

Hemophilia

One well-known example of an X-linked disorder is hemophilia. For this disorder, in which blood does not clot properly, there is a blood test that can identify carriers with about 90 percent accuracy.

Muscular dystrophy

Certain forms of muscular dystrophy, in which progressive deterioration of muscles leads to crippling and early death, also are X-linked disorders. A blood test with about 75 percent accuracy can indicate if a woman is a carrier of this disease. There are a number of other carrier tests for MD, including the recently developed ribosomal protein synthesis test, which some experts believe can identify carriers much more accurately than the blood test. Faulty protein synthesis has been found in the muscles of muscular dystrophy victims. Using a sample of the woman's muscle, the ribosomal protein synthesis test determines whether proteins are being manufactured in sufficient quantity.

Multifactorial diseases

Multifactorial, or polygenic, disorders spring not from a single altered gene or chromosome but from many genes acting together and with such factors as the environment.

Spina bifida

Spina bifida—a type of neural tube defect—is one such multifactorial genetic disorder, affecting about six thousand American newborns each year. Though there are three types of spina bifida, basically the defect occurs because the spinal column develops improperly in early pregnancy. Corrective surgery soon after birth is often necessary to save an infant with severe spina bifida. Those who survive may suffer brain damage, mental retardation, paralysis of the legs, and lack of bowel and bladder control. It is not possible to predict before a pregnancy who may bear a child with a multifactorial disease such as spina bifida unless the parents or other relatives also have the disorder, or a child has already been born with the disease. An increasing number of such disorders may be identified in the fetus through an amniocentesis done during pregnancy (for a more complete discussion of amniocentesis see page 52).

Infections

Besides genes, certain infections in the mother may cause birth defects in the fetus. For some of these infections, tests can now be administered before pregnancy to determine whether a woman already has an immunity (perhaps as a child she had the disease). If she is not immune and the disease is a serious possibility, she can be vaccinated before pregnancy. She cannot be vaccinated while pregnant.

Rubella

Rubella, or German measles, is among the deadliest of teratogenic infections. The disease in the mother may be relatively mild, involving no more than a sore throat, a slight rash, and a brief, low-grade fever. However, rubella can cause fetal death, deafness, blindness, or mental retardation, especially if the mother contracts the disease during the first twelve weeks of pregnancy. During the famous rubella epidemic of 1964–65, fifty thousand American infants were stillborn or deformed because their mothers caught the disease early in their pregnancies. Although a vaccine for protection against rubella was licensed in 1969, many women of childbearing age have never been vaccinated and are unsure if they are immune.

If you want to start a family, even in the distant future, and you are not certain whether you ever had rubella or were vaccinated for it, your doctor can determine this with a simple blood test. Should the test show no immunity or a low level, it's probably best to be vaccinated as soon as possible—if you are not pregnant and do not plan to be so for at least the next three months. If you *are* pregnant and have no immunity, you might, if at all possible, limit your contact with school-age children, who are likely carriers, during the first three months of pregnancy.

Toxoplasmosis

Toxoplasmosis (tahk-suh-plaz-mo'-suhs)—a relatively minor illness—may have catastrophic effects on a fetus. Parasites are transmitted primarily in raw or undercooked meat, or in the feces of infected cats. Like rubella, toxoplasmosis is mild enough in most individuals—something like a cold or flu with swollen glands. But when the disease strikes expectant mothers, or women just before they become pregnant, the fetus may suffer death, premature birth, or eye or brain damage. If you have had a history of toxo-plasmosis, or borne a child affected by the disease, your physician will probably order a blood test to determine if you are now im-mune. Once your immunity is verified, you cannot pass the disease on to any babies you may later bear. Unfortunately, no vaccine is yet available to prevent the disease. Pregnant women should avoid cats—especially their litter pans—and consume only thoroughly cooked meats.

Cytomegalovirus

Cytomegalovirus (syt-uh-meg-uh-lo-vy'-ruhs), or CMV, is another infection that may cause mild flulike symptoms in the mother but be disastrous for the fetus. More than 50 percent of women of childbearing age evidence previous exposure to CMV. The infection may be spread through tears, saliva, urine, endocer-vical mucous, semen, or any mucous membrane secretion. Some effects of CMV on the fetus include mental retardation, blindness, deafness, and liver and heart disorders. No vaccine has yet been developed to inoculate women against CMV. But blood tests are available to inform a woman before she conceives if she is immune to the infection.

Sexually transmitted disease

Venereal, or sexually transmitted, disease is one of America's most serious and fastest-spreading health problems. It is estimated that some 8.5 million Americans experienced some form of VD in 1977. While venereal disease is alarming for anyone who contracts it, the disease can be especially harmful to the developing fetus. If you are contemplating a pregnancy, don't wait until you conceive for a VD test or cure. If you suspect you have been infected, visit a doctor or public health officer immediately.

Syphilis

When syphilis is passed from mother to fetus, the bacteria may cause death, blindness, and other severe organic and tissue damage in the child. It was formerly believed that the syphilis spi-rochetes (spy'-ruh-keets), or bacteria, could not cross the placenta until after the twentieth week of pregnancy, but recent studies in-dicate that this can occur at any time. Some syphilis-related dis-orders may not surface until the infant is a teenager or young adult.

A blood test will determine the presence of syphilis; it is done routinely on pregnant women during one of their first prenatal visits, and again during the last weeks of pregnancy. If the initial blood test is positive, the doctor will most likely order another type of blood test for syphilis for further, more specific evaluation. Usually the disease can be quickly cured with penicillin.

Gonorrhea

Gonorrhea most often attacks the eyes of babies as they move through the infected birth canal. To prevent blindness due to gonorrheal infection, all states require that silver nitrate or penicillin drops be put in the newborn's eyes. Doctors sometimes detect gonorrhea in women by microscopic examination of a slide smeared with discharge from the cervix, vagina, rectum or other area. More reliable, though, is the culture test, in which a smear of discharge is incubated in a lab to allow gonorrheal bacteria to appear. Large doses of antibiotics, usually penicillin, will cure the infection promptly.

Herpesvirus type 2

Herpesvirus type 2, another sexually transmitted disease, causes sores on the genitals and is associated with miscarriage, prematurity, and low birth weight when it is contracted by a pregnant woman. The virus can also be transmitted from mother to baby during delivery, and infected newborns may display some mental or physical damage. No complete cure exists for herpesvirus type 2, although doctors can help control the disease. A pregnant woman with herpes may have to undergo a cesarean section to prevent her baby from contracting the infection. Confirming tests for herpes are a serum test for antibodies and a microscopic examination of a smear taken from a sore or from the cervix.

Group B strep

The group B streptococcus is a bacterium that may live in the genital tract of some women without causing specific symptoms, but infect a baby during delivery. If the infant contracts the "early-onset" type of group B strep infection, he or she may be premature, experience breathing problems, and suffer spinal meningitis, brain damage, and, frequently, death. "Late-onset" infections begin a week to a few months after birth and cause spinal meningitis, some brain damage, and—in 20 percent of the cases—death. Though penicillin sometimes helps cure the disease, there is no way to prevent it. Nor is there any test to determine if a woman is immune to the infection. Some doctors, however, take vaginal cultures periodically during pregnancy to learn if a woman has B strep, treat her, and thus try to prevent problems for the infant.

Nongonococcal urethritis

Nongonococcal urethritis (NGU) has received increasing attention lately as being the most common type of sexually transmitted disease. Though the infection often seems to be caused by the bacteria responsible for gonorrhea, NGU is mainly caused by the bacterium *Chlamydia trachomatis.* Some women experience no symptoms of NGU, while others have infections of the cervix or other pelvic areas. Infants may pick up the disease as they pass through the birth canal, and then suffer pneumonia and eye infections. Physicians usually diagnose the disease by first examining a culture or smear for gonococcal bacteria. If none exists, *Chlamydia* is the suspected source of trouble and the infection is treated with erythromycin or tetracycline.

Diabetes

Many other diseases that women suffer may have special effects on their pregnancies. In the past, for example, diabetics who became pregnant risked their own lives and the lives of their infants. Diabetics have an abnormally high level of sugar in their blood and urine, caused by a lack of insulin, a hormone produced by the pancreas. This insulin deficiency seriously upsets body chemistry. The demands of a pregnancy and fetus further disturb the body's balance and may intensify the disease. Before synthetic insulin was developed, about one-fourth of diabetic women who became pregnant died, and more than half the babies born of diabetic women died. With the advent of synthetic insulin in 1921, diabetics could stabilize the disease and meet the demands of pregnancy. However, there are still many medical concerns, such as the potential for increased birth defects, associated with pregnancy and diabetes. Today, women who determine that they have diabetes (through tests for sugar in their blood and urine), and control the disease before conception, have a better chance of producing healthy children.

In addition, about 1 percent of all pregnant women, with no prior history of diabetes, develop the disease *during* pregnancy. These women require careful prenatal monitoring and will probably see their doctors frequently during pregnancy.

Tests during pregnancy

Even during the most normal pregnancy, a woman undergoes many tests to evaluate her health. Anyone who's had prenatal care well remembers the routine of checking weight gain and blood pressure, taking a blood sample and urine specimen. These are all simple ways of telling how a woman's body is reacting to the changes brought on by pregnancy. In addition, in recent years pregnant women have undergone many more sophisticated tests that can accurately determine the health of their unborn children.

Rh blood factors

One of the first tests a woman receives as part of her prenatal care involves taking a sample of her blood to learn her major blood type and Rh factor. As we mention in Chapter 4 (see page 67), knowing whether a woman and the father of her child have Rh-positive or Rh-negative blood is extremely important to the health of the baby.

If the potential for an Rh problem exists, you'll have another blood test early in pregnancy to determine if any antibodies are present in your blood. If they are present, you'll probably have blood tests regularly during pregnancy to monitor the degree of this sensitization. When a certain level of sensitization is reached, your doctor will learn how affected your baby is by performing an amniocentesis (see below for a description of this procedure). Some doctors may opt to use a series of amniocenteses, rather than maternal blood tests, to monitor the baby's condition.

Depending on health and maturity, the fetus may: (1) be allowed to go full term, then receive transfusions of healthy blood; (2) be delivered a few weeks early; (3) receive healthy red blood cells while still in the uterus. If your initial blood screening shows no antibodies, you will deliver at term and receive an injection of anti-Rh gamma globulin (Rhogam) to prevent sensitization. This injection should be administered to Rh-negative women within seventy-two hours of each delivery. If antibodies show up later in pregnancy, an amniocentesis will probably be done, and the three options described above are available.

Amniocentesis

Amniocentesis (am-nee-o-sen-tee'-suhs) is a prenatal test that most women have heard about and an increasing number undergo every year (though many specialists feel that many women who *should* have amniocentesis do not). Basically, amniocentesis is the withdrawal of a small amount of the amniotic fluid, which surrounds and protects the baby in the uterus. This fluid contains cells from the fetal skin, mouth, urine, and intestinal tract, which usually can be cultured in a laboratory. After a certain stage of growth is reached in the lab, the cells are analyzed. This amniotic fluid reveals a remarkable amount of data about fetal health. It may indicate, for example, whether the fetus is being harmed by Rh incompatibility.

Another—and probably the best-known—use of the procedure is to detect genetic disorders early in pregnancy. Several hundred such disorders are now detectable through amniocentesis, including all chromosomal problems, such as Down's syndrome; biochemical abnormalities, such as Tay-Sachs disease; and neural tube defects, such as spina bifida (detectable by measuring the amount of a substance called alpha-fetoprotein in the amniotic fluid). As for X-linked disorders that are inherited through the sex chromosomes (see page 45), at present only a handful can be specifically identified in the fetus by examining the amniotic fluid. For the almost two hundred other X-linked diseases, the only alternative is to determine the sex of the fetus—easily done by means of amniocentesis. For example, genetic studies may indicate to a couple that there is a history of an X-linked disease, such as hemophilia, in their family. This disease strikes only males, and there is a 50 percent chance that each male conceived will have the disorder. In such a case, if the parents learn through amniocentesis that the fetus is male, they may opt to terminate the pregnancy. But the picture for hemophilia carriers may be changing; see the section on fetoscopy, below.

To determine genetic defects, amniocentesis is optimally performed at fourteen to sixteen weeks of pregnancy, when enough amniotic fluid has been produced to allow removal of a sampling for analysis. You may have the procedure done in your doctor's office, or in a hospital as an outpatient, and it may include genetic counseling. Usually, before an amniocentesis is performed, a doctor will locate the position of the fetus and placenta, and determine fetal age more precisely with an ultrasound scan (see page 55).

Another use of amniocentesis, besides revealing birth defects, is to determine fetal lung maturity, a vital consideration if a deliv-

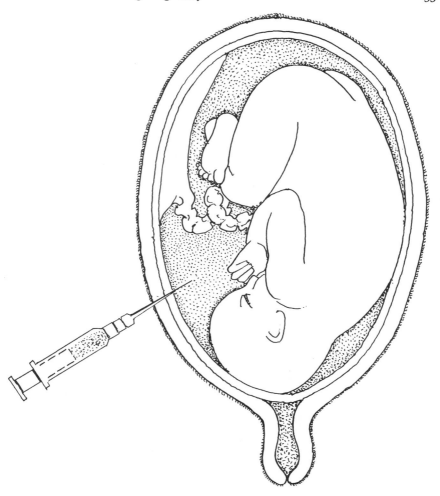

Fig. 13. Amniocentesis

ery (usually by cesarean section) must be done before term. Lung maturity can be determined by measuring the amounts of two substances, lecithin and sphingomyelin, found in the amniotic fluid. When the ratio of lecithin to sphingomyelin is at least 2 to 1 (usually after the thirty-fifth week of pregnancy), the baby's lungs will be able to function properly outside the uterus.

The procedure

For the amniocentesis, the woman is draped, a portion of her abdomen swabbed with antiseptic, and then a small amount of local anesthetic may be injected into the abdomen. (Some doctors forgo this injection, feeling it causes more discomfort than the amniocentesis needle.) After this, a longer, thin needle is injected through the abdomen into the uterus, and the amniotic fluid is withdrawn. The desired amount of fluid is placed in vials for lab analysis, and a small bandage is used to cover the puncture site. The procedure usually takes only a few minutes. Most women report minimal pain and pressure, or none at all, and do not need to change their routine after the exam.

Unfortunately, fluid cannot be withdrawn on the first try in all of the taps. In about 10 percent of the cases, the initial tap does not yield cells that can be cultured, and the procedure must be repeated. Such a delay can be frustrating for a couple who wish to learn as soon as possible about the fetus's health. Another source of anxiety is the waiting period—three to four weeks—while the cells are grown and analyzed. Many women experience feelings of helplessness and ambivalence during that time, when they may be uncertain if they will continue the pregnancy. For more than 95 percent of those tested, though, the result of the amniocentesis is good news—no disorders are found. These women can continue the pregnancy without the worry that their child may be born with defects.

In addition, for some diseases detected early, amniocentesis can mean early treatment to save the fetus. For example, if the fetus suffers from galactosemia (guh-lak-tuh-see'-mee-uh), an inability to digest milk products, placing the mother on a special prenatal diet can prevent organic damage, mental retardation, or the death of the baby.

Indications for amniocentesis

Who, then, should have amniocentesis for genetic disorders, and what are the risks involved? Generally, specialists feel amniocentesis is indicated if one (or more) of the following conditions exists:

1. The mother is thirty-five or older. Studies have shown that the chances of a woman producing a child with a chromosomal disorder increase after age thirty-five. This may happen because the eggs, present in the mother's body before her own birth, begin

to deteriorate with age or are subject to greater doses of dangerous elements such as radiation or chemicals the older she gets. Some experts feel that sperm may be similarly affected if the father is older than fifty-five, and may suggest amniocentesis for this reason.

2. A previous pregnancy produced a child with a chromosomal abnormality or an inheritable disease that can be diagnosed prenatally.

3. Either parent is known or thought to be a carrier of a chromosomal abnormality or inheritable disease.

Safety of amniocentesis

In recent years, many studies have been done to determine the safety of amniocentesis for the fetus and mother. Generally, the procedure seems to be very safe. Maternal problems are minor: a small number of women studied report passing cramps, some spotting, or slight leakage of amniotic fluid. But there is a slight risk that amniocentesis may precipitate abortion. Most studies peg this risk at less than 1 percent. Other fetal problems include puncture and premature delivery, but these appear to be rare occurrences.

Fetoscopy

At present, this is an experimental procedure. Employing a fiberoptic device inserted through the mother's abdomen, the physician determines the position of fetal blood vessels at the placental site. A minute quantity of blood is removed, then analyzed. Hemophilia, sickle-cell anemia, and thalassemia can be detected by means of this procedure, and there is hope that many more disorders will be diagnosable using this technique.

Ultrasound

The use of ultrasound waves is another way of learning about the fetus. Many obstetricians feel ultrasound exams should and will become a standard part of prenatal care. Other experts view routine ultrasound as overly interventionistic and unnecessary for normal pregnancies. The fact remains that more women are undergoing this exam, usually in their doctor's office or in a hospital unit. Before the development of ultrasound for obstetric purposes, physicians had to rely on X rays to reveal necessary information about the fetus. However, the potential dangers of direct radiation on the fetus have reduced the use of X rays as a diagnostic tool during pregnancy. Ultrasound, though, appears to be safe for mother and baby.

Ultrasonic exams involve externally directing high-frequency sound waves at the uterine area. When the waves bounce off the tissues in that area, they produce an image of the fetus and placenta on a small TV-like screen, and can be photographed for a permanent record. When the doctor or technician looks at these images, s/he can gain important information, such as an estimate of fetal size and age (determined by measurement of the fetal head); the position and condition of the fetus and placenta (vital for amniocentesis); whether any structural abnormalities exist in the fetal head; and if more than one fetus is present. Today, ultrasound can even inform women who appear to be miscarrying if the pregnancy will abort or if it has a good chance of survival.

Ultrasound exams are painless and should take only a few minutes. For the procedure, women are directed to have a full bladder, which is used as a guidepost when viewing the images on the screen. The exam room is darkened, and the woman lies supine on an examining table with the ultrasound machine nearby. The doctor applies a gel or other lubricant to the woman's uncovered abdomen, then moves a small, boxlike instrument around that area. Eventually, a clear image of the fetus and placenta will register on the small screen of the machine. The doctor may point out significant structures and organs, then photograph certain "shots" for the records.

Estriol tests

The measurement of estriol excretion in a pregnant woman's urine is another method of judging fetal health. Estriol is one of the principal estrogens that the placenta and fetus produce in increasing amounts during a pregnancy, and it is excreted into the urine. The level of urinary estriol will indicate the well-being of the fetal-placental unit. The test is especially important when the mother is suffering from toxemia, hypertension, or diabetes, or if the fetus is thought to be postmature. To measure estriol, a pregnant woman collects all her urine in one container over a twenty-four-hour period. The testing should be done at least twice within about a one-week period to have a standard for measurement, and may be done regularly if other conditions, such as diabetes, warrant it. Though the procedure is painless, it can be inconvenient.

Stress tests

If the physician suspects the placenta may not be functioning properly (because of toxemia, diabetes, kidney disease, or hypertension, for example) or that the fetus may be in danger, a woman may undergo a "stress test" near the end of pregnancy. The results of this test are used to decide whether the fetus is doing well enough to remain within the uterus and then undergo labor and delivery at a later date, or whether labor should be induced or a cesarean section performed soon to halt fetal distress.

This stress test, also called the oxytocin challenge test, is administered in a hospital, with the woman resting in bed. Initially, an external fetal monitor (see page 266) is attached to the patient, and fetal heart rate and uterine contractions are observed for about a half hour. This "non-stress-test" portion of the exam may constitute the entire test if the heart rate and contractions are shown to be normal. If an abnormal condition appears, the woman begins to receive increasing amounts of the hormone oxytocin (or pitocin) until it causes three uterine contractions, lasting forty to sixty seconds each, within a ten-minute period. When this is achieved, the contractions and fetal heart rate are carefully monitored for about thirty minutes.

The induced contractions are usually painless, similar in sensation to Braxton-Hicks contractions (see page 255). If the results of the test are satisfactory, the fetus can safely stay in the uterus for at least another week, when the mother will probably be tested again if the time is not right for delivery. If premature labor would definitely be hazardous for the fetus, or if the woman has undergone a previous cesarean section, the stress test would not be administered.

X-ray pelvimetry

Toward the end of pregnancy, X-ray measurement of the mother's pelvis may be necessary to determine whether vaginal delivery is possible, or whether the pelvis is too small to accommodate the baby's head and therefore cesarean surgery is indicated. X-ray pelvimetry may be performed during labor if the baby's head is not descending despite strong contractions and a well-dilated cervix.

CHAPTER FOUR
Common Discomforts and Complications

As you can see from the chart on page 14, every system in your body is affected by pregnancy: hormones released by the placenta act on the reproductive, respiratory, digestive, cardiovascular, nervous, and urinary systems. It's not surprising, then, that an array of physical discomforts and complaints reflect this widespread activity.

In many cases, problems can be minimized by rearranging activities, by exercising, by lying down, or by abstaining from certain foods. Drugs—over-the-counter or prescribed—should be a last resort. If a physician prescribes medication, *be sure s/he knows you are pregnant.* Double-check on that drug's safety with your obstetrician or nurse-midwife. If your obstetrician orders a drug for you, don't hesitate to question its necessity.

Common discomforts

•*Frequent urination.* Present during the first and third trimesters. In the first trimester, the blood vessels of the bladder are congested and the whole urinary system is sluggish. In the third trimester, these changes plus the weight of the baby on the bladder cause an everpresent urge to urinate, and sometimes a condition known as *stress incontinence*—the loss of urine during such stress as coughing or sneezing. Urination may be uncomfortable, incomplete, or even slightly irritating. To relieve discomforts, avoid caffeine, which is in coffee, tea, and soft drinks. Caffeine not only has a diuretic effect; it also increases bladder irritability. Some women say a warm bath or a hot-water bottle over the vulva relieves discomfort.

If you feel pressure on the bladder, a change in position may help. When you're lying on your side, support pillows under your abdomen may offer relief. *After* urinating, Kegel exercises (see page 158) may be beneficial because they help bring blood and oxygen to the urinary organs. Finally, to stave off nocturia (urinating at night), limit liquids after 6:00 P.M. If stress incontinence is a problem, wear a small panty shield. If you have a burning sensation or notice blood while urinating, call the doctor. You may have an infection. (During pregnancy many women begin a struggle with urinary infections that may last for years. In addition, women with urinary tract infections are more susceptible to pyelonephritis (pi-lo-ni-frit'-uhs), a common complication of pregnancy.)

• *Nausea.* Present during the first trimester and, rarely, into the second. Excessive vomiting may indicate a multiple pregnancy. Amazingly for such a common problem, little is known of its cause, although medical textbooks list HCG (the hormone detected in your urine during a pregnancy test), hormone imbalance, and changes in the digestive system as possible causes. Psychological factors may *trigger* nausea, but if you start blaming yourself for a condition you can't tolerate anyway, you'll only wind up feeling guilty. Instead, to combat nausea, keep some food in your stomach. Sustain blood-sugar levels by eating small high-protein or bland meals often; or snack in the midmorning, midafternoon, and before retiring. Some women find that they can eat only crackers, Zwieback and toast, mashed potatoes, and dry cereals. Other women cannot tolerate meats, dairy products, fried and greasy foods, or exotic dishes.

Cigarettes and alcohol, besides being harmful to your baby, may make you even more ill. The caffeine in coffee and the nicotine in cigarettes may stimulate an already irritated digestive system. Instead of coffee or tea, try unchilled carbonated beverages or even herbal teas.

For some women, strong smells start waves of nausea, and they find it better to stay in well-ventilated, smokeless rooms. Even too much cologne can be upsetting. Wearing loose-fitting clothes (try avoiding turtlenecks!) can help; and if you rinse with mouthwash or even water, or chew gum and suck on candies, your mouth will feel fresher.

Schedule activities around your queasy times; minimize morning activities if that's the time you're sickest; lie down when you can, or even stay in bed until you feel better. Try to avoid bending over if you must be up and around; don't wash your hair over the sink, and don't bend to wash your face or pick up a child (keep your back and head straight, then kneel). Have someone else do the bending part of cleaning, or forget about floors and tubs. Brushing your teeth can be postponed until morning queasiness has passed; some women use a mouthwash instead. And if vitamin pills have been prescribed but they make you gag, crush them between sheets of waxed paper and sprinkle the powder into applesauce or a mashed potato.

If these measures don't help, your physician may prescribe Bendectin, which works by relaxing the digestive system. The drug, unfortunately, may have unpleasant side effects, which the *Physicians' Desk Reference* lists as "drowsiness, vertigo, nervousness, epigastric pain, headache, palpitations, diarrhea, disorientations, and irritability." Some women recommend vitamin B_6 (pyridoxine hydrochloride). While this vitamin is important to maternal and fetal health, there is no hard evidence that it can stop nausea.

Finally, a word about nutrition. If nausea has caused a slight change in your diet, you may be concerned that the baby's nutritional needs are not being met. Don't be—*if* you have been well nourished all along. Eat what you can and the baby will get adequate nutrition from that and your body stores for approximately the first half of pregnancy.

•Fatigue. Primarily present during the first trimester and the last half of the third. Fatigue may be due to new hormonal patterns in the early stages; in the ninth month, it may be due to extra weight and loss of sleep because of discomfort and nocturia. Give in to the urge to sleep or nap when exhausted; otherwise, exercise moderately. Even though most of us feel the need—and sometimes the pressure—to be active and productive throughout pregnancy, it's important to tune into our bodies and do what feels natural. Sometimes just lying on the left side (a position that relieves pressure on blood vessels) for an hour can help; energizing yoga exercises, or those that get rid of tenseness, are good, too. Even if you can't arrange your day to accommodate too much more sleep, you can change positions, take walks, get fresh air, and keep strenuous sports to a minimum.

• Vaginal discharge. With changing hormone levels, the endocervical glands (glands inside the cervix) increase activity. The discharge is thick and white, with no odor. Douching won't help and could be dangerous; in any case, it can't stop the glands from secreting, and may increase the discharge. To avoid irritation, wear

small pads, cotton underpants, and looser slacks for comfort. Frequent showering or bathing will help you feel less sticky (but avoid medicated or perfumed soaps, which might be irritating). Talcum powder dusted on your thighs may help minimize chafing from the moisture, and you may avoid irritation by not wearing underpants at night. If you have a real problem controlling discharge, ask your doctor to examine you. If the discharge gets thick and foamy, or if your vulva itches, you may have contracted a mild infection, such as the following:

Candida albicans causes an itchy feeling and sometimes vaginal swelling. Your physician may prescribe a fungicide, such as Mycostatin or Monistat.

Trichomonas vaginalis may cause a foamy discharge, also with itching. Flagyl is often prescribed, but some studies have indicated that under certain conditions this drug may cause cancer in laboratory mice. In any case, Flagyl can cross the placenta and is contraindicated for pregnant women.

Nonspecific vaginitis is an infection of unknown cause. Bubble baths and deodorants may increase irritation. The infection may respond to sulfa creams.

•*Nosebleeds and stuffy nose.* The inside of the nose may become swollen and congested during pregnancy. You'll feel stuffy and your nose may run, but it's generally not good to use nosedrops, which, after giving relief, may actually increase swelling. If you irritate your nose excessively when you clear it, you may get a nosebleed.

Vaseline on the membranes can lubricate, and pinching can stop bleeding. If stuffiness is a problem, lean (not too close) over a pot of steaming, minted water, with a towel over your head to hold in the steam. Increase the humidity in your house or apartment by using a humidifier or vaporizer (for a real problem, you can run a steaming shower and sit in the bathroom for a while). For sleeping, raise the head of your bed (with wooden blocks under the legs). Avoid blowing your nose too hard, and keep your hands away from your nose.

•*Constipation.* Present during the first and third trimesters. Generally the hormonal changes of pregnancy slow down the digestive tract. Crowding of the intestines by the enlarging uterus makes matters worse. Slower movement of food through the large bowel may mean increased absorption of water, making feces dry. The important thing is to get liquids into your system (yes, you will be urinating even more, but that probably will feel better, too, because you'll be urinating with a full bladder). Drink lots of fluids (prune juice is good), eat vegetables and fruit (even dried fruit) for bulk, take mineral oil, and avoid constipating foods, such as rice, cheese, and chocolate. Sometimes, during the last months, because of separation of the recti muscles (the vertical muscles that corset the trunk), bearing down for a bowel movement is difficult. Try wrapping your arms around your stomach and bringing muscles together while you bear down. Also, bear down intermittently and gently.

Sometimes the problem is psychological. You feel you should have a bowel movement every day, but you can't. Some women suggest trying to defecate at the same time every day while relaxing with a good book. Others say that this "timing" makes them even more tense. In any case, exercise (some yoga postures are specifically designed to aid the bowels), a good diet, and relaxed visits to the bathroom do help. Don't self-medicate with suppositories, laxatives or enemas.

• **Hemorrhoids.** Like other veins in the lower portion of the body, the rectal veins dilate and experience increased pressure during pregnancy. If you're constipated and you strain to move your bowels, swollen veins may protrude through the rectum. To minimize hemorrhoids, avoid constipation. Cotton soaked in witch hazel and applied to the rectum, ice, Preparation H, and Vaseline may all help. When you move your bowels, use Tucks pads to clean yourself, or try soft toilet paper moistened with water. Sitting on hard chairs may help, too, and lying with your feet elevated will minimize pressure on anal veins.

• **Swelling** (edema). Present in the last trimester. As pressure on blood vessels increases, fluid is squeezed out to the surrounding tissues. Ankles, feet, and, to a lesser degree, hands and face get puffy. The swelling can be uncomfortable, but unless it's related to toxemia or kidney or heart disease, mild swelling is not dangerous. *It should never be treated with diuretics.* For relief, you can try lying on your left side for an hour in the morning and afternoon (*postural diuresis,* as this is known, will decrease pressure on major veins and allow blood to flow back to the heart more easily). If you can't lie down, put your feet up. Remove constricting clothes, such as knee socks with elastic tops, or rings, or watches. Cold water, astringent on your face, or air conditioning may make you feel better but won't decrease edema. Don't attempt to cut down on liquids or salt. You need both, and any limitation, without the advice of someone knowledgeable, can actually make swelling worse and subject your system to dangerous stress.

• *Excessive salivation* (ptyalism [ti'-uh-liz-uhm]). Present during the entire pregnancy, this complaint is rare but very aggravating. Saliva floods the mouth, but more annoying is the acrid taste that accompanies the saliva. Mouthwash, gum, and mints will keep your mouth fresh; even rinsing your mouth with water will get the bad taste out. Frequent small meals will help. Suck on a lemon wedge, brush teeth often, and sleep with a glass of water and an empty bowl by the bed so that you can rinse during the night. Unfortunately, no medication will offer consistent relief.

• *Backache and frontache.* Present during the first and third trimesters. During pregnancy, the pelvic joints in front and the sacroiliac joints in back relax in anticipation of delivery. In addition to the strains this causes, your expanding uterus forces you to curve your back inward for balance, further tiring and straining muscles. The results may be aching in front and in back, sometimes to the extent that walking becomes uncomfortable. For backache, the pelvic rock is excellent (for a description of this exercise, see page 158). With practice, you can do the pelvic rock while standing— even on a train or bus.

Heat, massage, sleeping on your side with legs spread as if you were running—all may help. Stick to straight-backed chairs and lower heels. Gym shoes and crepe-soled shoes feel great, too. Wearing a girdle may give relief in extreme cases of muscle laxity, but a girdle will not build up the muscles needed for support.

• *Shortness of breath.* Present during the third trimester. As the baby grows, the uterus pushes the diaphragm up, diminishing your lung capacity. As soon as the baby "drops," leaving more room for the diaphragm, the problem lessens. Until that time, fresh air and well-ventilated rooms are preferable. Try taking deep, slow breaths through the mouth; rest; don't overexert; and minimize running up steps. Loose clothes on chest and stomach may help; but tight-fitting collars and jewelry, as well as tight, Empire-style maternity dresses may make you feel constricted. Always stand up straight to allow plenty of room for lungs to expand. Above all, don't get upset about shortness of breath. If you do, you might begin to hyperventilate (this can be cured by breathing into your cupped hands or a paper bag).

• *Leg cramps.* Present during the third trimester. Nobody really knows what causes leg cramps, although you may hear that you should decrease your milk intake to cut down on phosphorus, increase your milk intake to get more calcium, increase salt, or double your prenatal vitamin dose. *Before you make any dietary change, consult your physician.* The best relief for leg cramps is to bend the foot in the opposite direction and massage; when you feel a cramp coming on, you can try flexing and extending your toes and arcing them in circles, or lie down and press your feet against the wall. Massage, heating pads, warm baths, and support hose all help, too. Women who wear grip-type shoes during pregnancy may have cramps more frequently. The gripping may set off muscle spasms. Generally, more supportive shoes will minimize cramping. Another remedy is propping your legs, as well as moving around, instead of standing or sitting in one position for too long. Moderate bicycling, walking, and swimming are good exercises. In the winter, wear leg warmers.

• *Heartburn.* Present from the first trimester through the third. The conventional wisdom has it that when you're pregnant your stomach produces more acid. This isn't true. The heartburn is caused by acid "splashing up" from the stomach to the esophagus. To minimize splashing, don't lie down after eating. To make your stomach act as efficiently as possible, eat light, frequent meals during the day instead of three large ones. Avoid heavy meals late at night that will take a long time to digest, and stay away from spicy and greasy foods. Once in a while, you can take Tums, Maalox, Gelusil, Rolaids, or Alka-Seltzer, although some doctors recommend avoiding these medications during the third trimester.

• *Varicose veins.* Present from the first trimester through the third. Because the growing uterus blocks the return of blood to the heart, blood is apt to "pool" in the legs. The pooled blood expands the veins, and they become visible and raised under the skin. The veins may make your legs feel heavy. If you still have varicose veins after pregnancy, they can be "stripped," or removed, but during pregnancy there's not much you can do except lie down frequently with your feet slightly elevated. Some women say that running and walking help by aiding the flow of blood. Support hose is often beneficial as well.

Complications of pregnancy

Almost any illness that occurs in nonpregnant women occurs in pregnant women, too. Illnesses must be treated carefully, with consideration for the developing embryo or fetus. In addition, some women encounter complications brought on by the pregnancy itself.

If your physician indicates that any of the following conditions (or anything else!) may be a problem, and you are interested in its causes and treatment, do some reading in such texts as *Williams Obstetrics* or the *American Journal of Obstetrics and Gynecology* (indexed to make it easier to find articles). They can be obtained from university medical libraries, and sometimes local libraries, or from childbirth groups in your community. The texts may be difficult, but they are not impossible to read.

• *Toxemia (preeclampsia, eclampsia).* High blood pressure, protein in the urine, rapid weight gain, excessive retention of fluid (edema), headaches, and visual disturbances characterize preeclampsia—the early stage of toxemia. Toxemia is usually associated with first pregnancies and may be more prevalent in women with high blood pressure, with kidney disease or diabetes, or women in poor health. Some doctors feel that poor nutrition plays a major role in the illness. Preeclampsia appears later in pregnancy and if untreated can lead to convulsions and coma, with great danger to baby and mother. This convulsive stage is called eclampsia. For preeclampsia, the best treatment is delivery of the baby if it is mature. When the fetus is not mature and should not be delivered, bed rest and an adequate, balanced diet are prescribed. In the patient with eclampsia, hospitalization, treatment with drugs, and careful monitoring of the mother are necessary until the fetus is mature enough to be delivered.

• *Ectopic pregnancy.* An ectopic pregnancy occurs when the fertilized egg implants outside the uterine cavity. The implantation site may be the Fallopian tubes, ovaries, abdomen, or cervix, although tubal pregnancies are most common. Tubal pregnancies may be caused by damage to the Fallopian tubes through illness, and are characterized by menstrual irregularity and abdominal pain caused by internal bleeding. Your doctor may detect a soft, tender pelvic mass. The fetus almost never survives to term. Instead, the tube may rupture. Surgery to remove it (and sometimes the ovary on the side of the affected tube) may be necessary. Early diagnosis of ectopic pregnancy is crucial.

•*Spontaneous abortion* (also called miscarriage). Some physicians define miscarriage as a pregnancy that ends, with no interference, before the twentieth week. Others define it as producing a fetus weighing less than five hundred grams (a little more than a pound); such a fetus is unlikely to be viable. As many as 20 percent of all known pregnancies end in spontaneous abortion. The cause may lie in the embryo: perhaps it had an abnormal chromosomal pattern that made life impossible, or perhaps the placenta could not sustain the embryo. Spontaneous abortion may also be the result of maternal problems, such as illness, accident, structural defects in the reproductive organs, insufficient or abnormal hormone production. Generally, a miscarriage begins with vaginal bleeding and cramping, although only half of all women experiencing these symptoms abort. There is no medication or regimen that will allow you to keep a pregnancy; by the time bleeding and cramping occur in most spontaneous abortions, the embryo has already died. In many cases the embryo is so malformed that survival would be impossible.

•*Multiple pregnancy.* About 1 percent of all births result in twins; about 0.015 percent result in triplets. Twins may be identical (if they're the result of one fertilized egg that splits) or fraternal (the product of two ova and two sperm). You may suspect you're pregnant with twins if your uterus seems unusually large or if nausea is particularly strong. Your physician may be able to feel two fetuses manually, or s/he may perform an ultrasound examination (or X ray if ultrasound is not available). The doctor may prescribe extra bed rest during the last trimester to prevent premature labor and also ask that you discontinue sexual relations. Generally, a woman pregnant with more than one child experiences all the usual discomforts of pregnancy—but to a greater degree.

•*Hydatidiform mole* (molar pregnancy). This cluster of grapelike tissue grows in the uterus and causes symptoms that mimic pregnancy: missed periods, nausea, enlarging uterus. Usually there is no fetus present, and the molar "pregnancy" ends at about the fourth month when the woman expels this tissue spontaneously. This condition is very rare, and a very small percentage of those women who have experienced it may develop a malignant growth. A molar pregnancy may delay, but does not prevent, future normal pregnancies.

• *Rh and other blood factors causing erythroblastosis.* Almost 90 percent of all Americans carry a substance in their blood called the Rh factor. The other 10 percent, considered "Rh negative," lack that component. Problems for pregnant women may arise if their blood is Rh negative and the fetus they carry is Rh positive (genetically possible because the father may carry the Rh-positive gene). The "negative" mother may build up antibodies against the blood of her "positive" fetus, resulting in anemia or even death to the fetus (erythroblastosis [i-rith-ruh-blas-to'-suhs]). These conditions are most likely to arise in second and later pregnancies.

Today, physicians can run prenatal tests to determine if a mother's blood contains antibodies. Also, they can give an injection of human anti-Rh gamma globulin (Rhogam) soon after delivery to Rh-negative, unsensitized mothers with "positive" babies, to prevent this buildup of antibodies.

Less dangerous, but sometimes a problem, is ABO incompatibility. At present there is no method that can be used prenatally to detect the incompatibility conclusively. A mother with type O blood may form antibodies that can attack the blood of her fetus if the fetus has type A or type B blood. These cases are rarely damaging to the fetus, although sometimes the infant develops jaundice after birth.

There are many other blood factors that can cause erythroblastosis in the fetus. If the cases are severe, intrauterine and postnatal blood transfusions may be performed.

CHAPTER FIVE
Staying Healthy to Keep Your Baby Healthy

Whatever you eat during pregnancy has a profound effect on your health and on that of your baby. Though this *seems* obvious, it's taken a while for many people, experts included, to see the connection between eating well during pregnancy and bearing a healthy child. Even today, not everyone understands the implications of good prenatal nutrition. For many, eating during pregnancy means only how much weight the mother gains.

In another era, pregnant women were counseled to "eat for two"—advice that may have added pounds but did not ensure a healthful diet. Not too long ago, even slim women were told to restrict their calories and gain only a small amount of weight during pregnancy. In recent years, the dangers of routine prenatal weight restriction have become clear. But more important, we understand better that pregnant women *must* eat foods of good nutritional quality to provide the material vital for sound fetal development.

Weight gain

Strict weight restriction during pregnancy is a thing of the past, since many studies have tied miscarriage, stillbirth, and the dangers of low birth weight to insufficient maternal gain. Today, most doctors recommend twenty to thirty pounds gained gradually and steadily throughout pregnancy. (Figure 14 on page 69 illustrates the pattern of such a gain.) A sudden, unexplained increase one month, along with other symptoms such as high blood pressure, edema, and protein in the urine, may indicate preeclampsia (see page 65). But some experts, Dr. Tom Brewer for one, strongly believe that if a pregnant woman eats quality foods, it doesn't matter how much weight she gains.

Patient's Name:_____

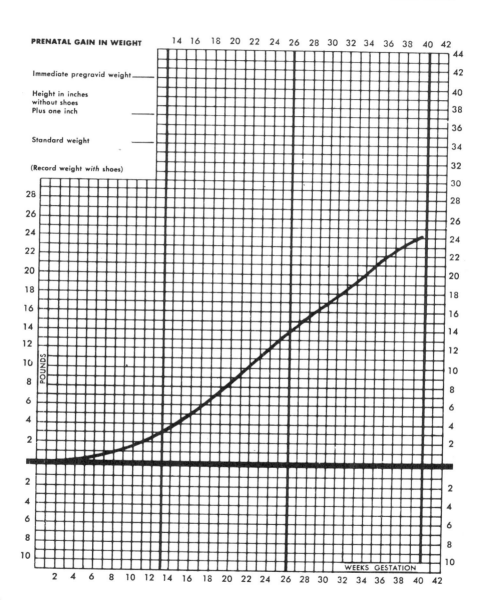

Fig. 14. Prenatal Weight Gain Grid

In the past, weight gain was a major concern because experts believed that limiting weight during pregnancy prevented toxemia (see page 65) and also helped a woman have an easier labor and delivery because of the baby's smaller size. These theories were later discredited. Today, many pregnant women say their doctors still impose a weight limit, yet never discuss which kinds of foods are important to eat.

Eating nutritiously is more important than counting calories or adding up pounds each month. Any woman who's ever been made to feel guilty when she gained more than her "allotted" weight during pregnancy—even when she was eating wisely—can appreciate Brewer's philosophy. Most pregnant women don't mind the extra weight during pregnancy if they know it will help produce a healthy child. Pregnancy is not the time to worry about being thin. Strenuous dieting is not advisable because it can cause problems in a pregnant woman and the fetus. If you eat quality—not junk— foods, the weight you gain will probably be easier to lose after delivery.

Nutritional needs during pregnancy

Pregnancy is a normal physiological state that causes a certain amount of stress on the body's systems. A woman's heart and entire cardiovascular system work harder; her blood volume increases; hormone production is stepped up; her body retains more water; her breasts and uterus enlarge; her appetite increases; and she gains enough weight to support the developing fetus. All these changes take a considerable amount of nourishment.

Women can prepare for a healthy pregnancy by following healthy eating habits even *before* conception. But improving diet at any point during pregnancy will have a positive effect on the mother and fetus. Once she conceives, a woman should have about 300 more calories daily, which normally is about 15 percent of her prepregnancy food intake. The extra calories are needed to supply adequate nutrients to the fetus and to replenish the mother's nutrient stores.

• *Protein.* One of the most important nutrients a pregnant woman needs is protein. It is vital for tissue growth and for building hormones, enzymes, and antibodies, and regulating body fluids. Also, studies have shown that insufficient protein intake in the mother is related to prematurity, stillbirth, birth defects, and reduced birth weight. Some researchers think that high-protein diets reduce the incidence of toxemia.

The average pregnant woman needs at least 75 grams of protein every day, though many experts recommend much higher amounts. (To illustrate, there are 7 grams of protein in an ounce of meat; 2 grams of protein in a slice of bread; 8 grams of protein in a glass of milk.) Besides the quantity of protein in her diet, a pregnant woman should consider the quality of the protein she eats— that is, whether the protein is "complete" or "incomplete."

Proteins are made up of amino acids. A protein is called "complete" when it contains sufficient amounts of "essential" amino acids, and "incomplete" when one or more of these amino acids are missing or in short supply. "Essential" means the body must get the amino acid directly from food—it cannot build the amino acid from substances already in the body.

A pregnant woman, like every human being, needs food with all the essential amino acids present in order to make protein the body needs. Eggs, milk and milk products, meat, poultry, fish and seafood are complete protein foods. Incomplete protein foods, such as beans and peas, nuts, soybeans, whole grains and cereals, can be combined to supply all the amino acids necessary for complete protein.

A pregnant woman who abstains from meat can still get complete protein by eating enough fish, eggs, or dairy products. If she avoids animal products altogether, she must eat enough vegetable products to provide the complete protein her body and her baby need. Strict vegetarians may want to consult a nutritionist or physician to make sure their protein intake is adequate for pregnancy.

Important minerals during pregnancy

•*Iron.* Because of her increased blood volume, in addition to the demands of the fetus, a pregnant woman needs more iron, especially during the second and third trimesters. Without enough iron, she runs the risk of becoming anemic. Since it's hard to get the necessary amount of iron through diet, doctors usually recommend that a prenatal supplement of 30 to 60 milligrams of iron be taken daily during the second half of pregnancy. Still, a pregnant woman should eat foods rich in iron, such as meat, liver, eggs, whole-grain breads and cereals, wheat germ, dry beans and peas, and leafy green vegetables, such as collard greens and kale. Despite reports that liver may contain questionable amounts of pesticides and chemical residues, it is still recommended—in moderation—for pregnant women as a good source of iron and vitamins.

• *Calcium.* Since fetal bones and teeth are developing, calcium is needed in larger amounts during pregnancy than normally. This increased demand can usually be met through diet. However, vegetarians who do not drink milk or eat milk products—the best sources for calcium—may have difficulty ingesting sufficient amounts of the mineral and may need a supplement.

• *Sodium.* Table salt is the chief source of sodium in our diets. A pregnant woman needs sodium both because of her expanded blood volume and to ensure good nutrient transfer within her body. Today, expectant mothers are usually advised to salt their food to taste and so meet the body's demands for that mineral. Sodium intake during pregnancy has been a controversial subject. Low-salt diets used to be considered the answer to edema and toxemia, and some physicians routinely suggested limiting salt intake for healthy pregnant patients. Experts now believe that sodium restriction during pregnancy is not warranted unless the woman has high blood pressure or heart or kidney disease, and that, in fact, such restriction may be detrimental to the fetus.

• *Iodine.* To a pregnant woman, iodine is essential for the proper function of both her own and the fetus's thyroid gland. The thyroid affects physical and mental development, and when insufficient iodine is supplied to the gland, the fetus may not grow normally. If she uses iodized salt, a pregnant woman will be assured of getting the necessary amount of iodine.

Other important minerals during pregnancy are:

- phosphorus (available in meats, milk and other dairy products, whole-grain cereals and flours)
- magnesium (in leafy green vegetables, grains, nuts, dairy products, dry beans)
- zinc (in meats, eggs, milk and milk products, whole grains, dry beans, and nuts)

Vitamins

Pregnancy probably increases the need for all vitamins, though nobody really knows by how much. We do know that folic acid—a B vitamin—is the only vitamin that cannot be sufficiently supplied by increasing food intake. Folic-acid deficiency can cause a type of anemia during the last trimester. Some studies have also linked severe folic-acid deficiency to miscarriage and other pregnancy complications. Therefore, a daily supplement of 400 to 800 micrograms of this vitamin is usually recommended for pregnant women.

To make sure their patients get enough of *all* necessary vitamins and minerals, physicians often prescribe a special prenatal supplement. This supplement usually contains relatively large amounts of vitamin A; the B-complex vitamins: thiamin, riboflavin, niacin, B_6, B_{12}, and folic acid (folacin); vitamins C, D, and E; and the minerals iron, calcium, iodine, and magnesium. Many doctors prescribe this supplement for their patients as soon as they learn they're pregnant.

Some physicians prefer to wait until after the twelfth week of pregnancy because the effects of the vitamins and minerals during that crucial period of development are not fully known. Other doctors do not routinely recommend prenatal supplements (except for iron and folic acid) because they feel that normal diets will supply the necessary amounts. Still others recommend a regular multiple vitamin that has the appropriate amounts of iron and folic acid. If your doctor does prescribe the costlier prenatal supplement, you may want to ask if you can take a regular multiple vitamin instead. Regardless of whether your doctor prescribes a prenatal vitamin supplement, nutritious dietary patterns are essential.

Getting the essential vitamins in food

The following list includes the essential vitamins along with some of their food sources:

vitamin A: leafy green and yellow vegetables (broccoli, carrots, sweet potatoes, squash, tomatoes, greens, spinach), fruits (apricots, peaches, cantaloupe), liver, butter and margarine

thiamin: pork, kidneys, wheat germ, whole-grain breads and cereals, dry beans and peas, nuts, soybeans

riboflavin: liver, milk, eggs, cottage cheese, yogurt, fish

niacin: meats, poultry, fish, liver, peanuts, dry beans and peas, wheat germ

vitamin B_6: liver, meats, fish, milk, whole-grain breads and cereals, legumes

vitamin B$_{12}$: liver, meats, eggs, fish, milk—since vegetable products are almost totally lacking in B$_{12}$, vegetarians who eat no
animal foods should take the vitamin in a supplement

folic acid: leafy green and yellow vegetables, whole-grain breads
and cereals, dry beans and peas, nuts, liver, kidneys

vitamin C: citrus fruits and their juices, cantaloupe, tomatoes,
green peppers, broccoli, strawberries, cabbage

vitamin D: milk and dairy products, sunshine

vitamin E: whole-grain breads and cereals, wheat germ, vegetable oils

For all the foods we've mentioned that supply protein, vitamins, and minerals, what are the necessary amounts for a pregnant
woman? First, it might help to divide foods into different groups.
The California Department of Health has prepared a helpful guide
that classifies foods into six groups: (1) protein foods; (2) milk and
milk products; (3) grain products; (4) vitamin C–rich fruits and
vegetables; (5) leafy green vegetables; and (6) other fruits and vegetables. A pregnant woman can use Table 1, the Daily Food Guide,
below to see how many servings from each of these six groups she
needs each day. Then, by choosing foods included in these groups
(see Table 2, pages 75–79), she can specifically determine her diet.

Table 1.
DAILY FOOD GUIDE

Number of servings

Food Group	Non-pregnant Woman	Pregnant Woman	Lactating Woman
Protein foods (animal and vegetable) ..	3	4	4
Milk and milk products ...	3	4	5
Grain products	3	3	3
Vitamin C–rich fruits and vegetables	1	1	1
Leafy green vegetables	2	2	2
Other fruits and vegetables	1	1	1

Table 2.
FOOD GROUPS

PROTEIN FOODS include both animal and vegetable foods. Animal protein foods supply protein, iron, riboflavin, niacin, vitamins B_6 and B_{12}, phosphorus, zinc, and iodine. Vegetable protein foods supply protein, iron, thiamin, folacin, vitamins B_6 and E, phosphorus, magnesium, and zinc.

Animal protein foods:*

A serving is 2–3 oz. (60–90gm) cooked (boneless) of the following unless otherwise noted:

Bacon, 6 slices
Beef: ground, cube, roast, chop
Canned tuna, salmon, crab, etc., ½ cup
Cheese (See Milk)
Chitterlings (tripe)
Clams, 4 large or 9 small
Crab
Duck
Eggs, 2
Fish, fillet, steak
Fish sticks, breaded, 4
Frankfurters, 2
Hogmaws
Lamb: ground, cube, roast, chop
Lobster
Luncheon meat, 3 slices
Organ meats: liver, kidney, sweetbreads, heart, tongue
Oysters, 10–15 medium
Pig ears
Pig's feet
Pig snouts
Pork, ham: ground, roast, chop
Poultry: ground, roast
Rabbit
Sausage links, 4
Shrimp, scallops, 5–6 large
Spareribs, 6 medium ribs
Veal: ground, cube, roast, chop

---

* An alternate protein food is a combination of animal (70 percent) and vegetable (30 percent) protein foods. Most commonly used is a mixture of meat and textured vegetable protein (TVP). Such foods have the advantage of being more economical than 100 percent animal protein foods.

Vegetable protein foods:

A serving is 1 cup cooked unless otherwise stated.
Canned garbanzo, lima, kidney beans
Canned pork and beans
Dried beans and peas
Lentils
Nut butters, $1/4$ cup
Nuts, $1/2$ cup
Sunflower seeds, $1/2$ cup
Tofu (soybean curd)

MILK AND MILK PRODUCTS is an exchange group for foods containing calcium, phosphorus, vitamin D, and riboflavin. In addition, these foods supply protein, vitamins A, E, B_6, and B_{12}, magnesium, and zinc. For some people, milk and milk products serve as primary sources of protein in the diet.

A serving is 8 oz. (1 cup or 240cc) unless otherwise noted.
Cheese: hard and semisoft (except bleu, Camembert, and cream), $1\frac{1}{2}$ oz.
Cheese spread, 2 oz.
Cottage cheese, creamed, $1\frac{1}{3}$ cups
Cow's milk: whole, nonfat, low fat, nonfat dry reconstituted, buttermilk, chocolate milk, cocoa made with milk
Cream soups made with milk, 12 oz.
Evaporated milk, 3 oz.
Goat's milk (low B_{12} content)
Ice cream, $1\frac{1}{2}$ cups
Ice milk
Instant breakfast made with milk, 4 oz.
Liquid diet beverage, 5 oz.
Milkshake, commercial, 8 oz.
Puddings, custard (flan)
Soybean milk (low B_{12} content)
Yogurt

Note: Tofu is also a source of calcium; 1 cup tofu may be exchanged for one serving of the above foods.

GRAIN PRODUCTS supply thiamin, niacin, riboflavin, iron, phosphorus, and zinc. This exchange group is divided into two parts: whole-grain items, and enriched products. The enriched breads, cereals, and pastas provide significantly lower amounts of magnesium and zinc. For this reason, patients should be urged to choose whole-grain products.

Whole-grain items:
Brown rice, $\frac{1}{2}$ cup
Cereals, hot: oatmeal (rolled oats), rolled wheat, cracked wheat, wheat and malted barley, $\frac{1}{2}$ cup cooked
Cereals, ready-to-eat: puffed oats, shredded wheat, wheat flakes, granola, $\frac{3}{4}$ cup
Cracked and whole wheat bread, 1 slice
Wheat germ, 1 Tbsp.

Enriched breads, cereals, and pastas:
Note: California law requires that bread and bakery products be made with enriched flours. The following should comply with this requirement.

Bread, 1 slice (all other forms)
Cereals, hot: cream of wheat, cream of rice, farina, cornmeal, grits, $\frac{1}{2}$ cup
Cereals, ready-to-eat, $\frac{3}{4}$ cup
Cornbread, 1 piece (2 inches square)
Crackers, 4 (all kinds)
Macaroni, noodles, spaghetti, cooked, $\frac{1}{2}$ cup
Muffin, biscuit, dumpling, 1
Pancake, 1 medium
Rice, cooked, $\frac{1}{2}$ cup
Roll, bagel, 1
Tortilla, corn, 2
Tortilla, flour, 1 large
Waffle, 1 large

VITAMIN C–RICH FRUITS AND VEGETABLES supply ascorbic acid. Fresh, frozen, or canned forms may be used, although vitamin C content of canned products is lower.

Juices:
Orange, grapefruit, 4 oz.
Tomato, pineapple, 12 oz.
Fruit juices and drinks enriched with vitamic C, 6 oz.

Fruits:
Cantaloupe, $\frac{1}{2}$
Grapefruit, $\frac{1}{2}$
Guava, $\frac{1}{4}$ medium
Mango, 1 medium
Orange, 1 medium
Papaya, $\frac{1}{3}$ medium
Strawberries, $\frac{3}{4}$ cup
Tangerine, 2 small

Vegetables:
Bok choy, $\frac{3}{4}$ cup
Broccoli, 1 stalk
Brussels sprouts, 3–4
Cabbage, cooked, $1\frac{1}{3}$ cups
Cabbage, raw, $\frac{3}{4}$ cup
Cauliflower, raw or cooked, 1 cup
Greens: collard, kale, mustard, Swiss chard, turnip greens, $\frac{3}{4}$ cup
Peppers, chili, $\frac{3}{4}$ cup
Peppers: green, red, $\frac{1}{2}$ medium
Tomatoes, 2 medium
Watercress, $\frac{3}{4}$ cup

LEAFY GREEN VEGETABLES is an exchange group for folacin. In addition, these foods supply vitamins A, E, and B_6, riboflavin, iron, and magnesium.

A serving is 1 cup raw, or $\frac{3}{4}$ cup cooked.
Asparagus
Bok choy
Broccoli
Brussels sprouts
Cabbage
Dark leafy lettuce: chicory, endive, escarole, red leaf, romaine
Greens: beet, collard, kale, mustard, spinach
Swiss chard, turnip
Scallions
Watercress

OTHER FRUITS AND VEGETABLES include yellow fruits and vegetables which supply significant amounts of vitamin A. Vitamin A is also found in outstanding amounts in the leafy green vegetable group. Other fruits and vegetables also contribute varying amounts of B-complex vitamins, vitamin E, magnesium, zinc, and phosphorus.

A serving is ½ cup (fresh, frozen, or canned) unless otherwise indicated.

Vegetables:

Artichoke
Bamboo shoots
Bean sprouts: alfalfa, mung
Beet
Burdock root
Carrot
Cauliflower
Celery
Corn
Cucumber
Eggplant
Beans: green, wax
Hominy
Lettuce: head, Boston, Bibb

Mushrooms
Nori seaweed
Onion
Parsnip
Peas
Pea pods
Potato
Radishes
Summer squash
Sweet potato
Winter squash
Yam
Zucchini

Fruits:

Apple, 1 medium
Apricot, fresh, 1 large
Banana, 1 small
Berries
Cherries
Dates, 5
Figs, 2 large
Fruit cocktail
Grapes
Kumquats, 3
Nectarines, 2 medium
Peach, fresh, 1 medium
Pear, 1 medium
Persimmon, 1 small
Pineapple
Plums, 2 medium
Prunes, 4 (also significant iron source)
Pumpkin, ¼ cup
Raisins (also significant iron source)
Watermelon

Nausea and eating during pregnancy

Many women (about 50 percent in the United States) experience nausea during pregnancy. The symptoms of nausea range from mild to severe. Some women feel slightly queasy only on awakening. Others have such powerful nausea, with frequent vomiting, that it disrupts every aspect of their lives until it is controlled.

For these women, eating (and even looking at or smelling food) can become a major concern. Many are reluctant to eat because of the nausea and vomiting that follow each meal or snack. Other expectant mothers are repelled only by certain foods—such as coffee or meat—which they ordinarily enjoy. While the study of prenatal nausea has produced many theories—such as a deep-seated desire *not* to be pregnant—and remedies—such as herbal teas and vitamin B_6—the fact remains that nausea can make eating well during pregnancy much more difficult.

Coping with nausea

Women cope with this problem in a variety of ways. But it's important to remember that each person is different—what works for some may not help others. Some suggestions:

• If nausea during pregnancy is primarily a *morning* sickness, it may help to munch crackers or sip ginger ale until the feeling passes. Also, some women find if they let themselves vomit or have the "dry heaves" in the morning, and keep something in their stomach at all times, the nausea is controlled.

• When "morning sickness" is really an all-day illness, a pregnant woman should eat what she can and not force down foods that may be nutritious but are totally unpalatable to her.

• Keep in mind that nausea is worsened by going without food for too long. Try to eat something, even if it's only a small amount. Some foods that might be tolerated better than others include: crackers, dry toast, Zweiback, baked or boiled potatoes, noodles, rice, gelatin, bouillon, ginger ale, fruit juices, fish, seafood, and lean meats.

• Often, milk and milk products do not sit well during a bout of nausea. Spicy, fried, fatty, and rich foods may increase queasiness. Too much liquid, drunk all at once, or with a meal, may also be nauseating.

Fortunately, most cases of pregnancy nausea are short-lived, usually stopping by the end of the first trimester. It may also help to know that if the mother is well nourished, the fetus can survive on nutrient stores within her body until mid-pregnancy. This fact doesn't eliminate the need to try to eat nutritiously. But it may remove some of that pressure from women who are aggravated enough by nausea. (See Chapter Four for further suggestions on coping with nausea.)

Dangerous substances in food

Increasingly, pregnant women have become aware of reports that certain foods may be harmful to the fetus.

• *Mercury in fish.* Recent reports that many fish contained amounts of mercury judged unacceptable by the U.S. Food and Drug Administration caused considerable public concern. Pregnant women have additional reason to worry about this information. Mercury poisoning produces a variety of physical and mental problems—many quite severe—in the fetus, as the tragic events in Minimata, Japan, have shown (see page 224).

To minimize the possibility of ingesting questionable amounts of mercury, some experts believe pregnant women should have no more than three 4-ounce servings of fish a week. Also, choosing different brands and varieties of fish should help decrease the chances of eating too much of a high-mercury type.

• *Blighted potatoes.* A few years ago, studies by James H. Renwick, an English geneticist, suggested that pregnant women should be wary of the potatoes they eat. Renwick theorized that women who in early pregnancy eat potatoes blighted by mold run a greater risk of having babies with neural tube defects such as spina bifida. He recommended avoiding discolored potatoes, since the brown and black marks may signal blight. While Renwick's hypothesis has caused much discussion, his findings have not been substantiated.

• *Food additives and pesticide residues.* Each year, more scientific reports appear, detailing the health hazards of certain substances in our foods. Nitrates and nitrites, used in cured meats for flavor and color, and to prevent botulism, have been linked to cancer. Saccharin, a sweetening agent, has been shown to produce bladder cancer in test animals. Some obstetricians are recommending that their patients avoid saccharin entirely. Diethylstilbestrol (DES), a synthetic hormone put in cattle and poultry feed, also produces cancer in lab animals. The DES fed to cattle and poultry may remain in their tissues and organs (especially the liver) and eventually be eaten by humans and remain in *our* tissues. In addition, DES given to pregnant women in the 1940s, 1950s, and 1960s to prevent miscarriage, resulted in an increase of the incidence of vaginal cancer among the daughters of these women.

The potent pesticides used to control destructive insects and unwanted vegetation also invade the food we eat. Farm animals ingest pesticides in feed and grass; fish consume the poison when it is sprayed near streams and lakes. Ultimately, residues reach the body and remain there. Pesticides affect fruits and vegetables, too, though in much lower concentrations than in meat, fish, and dairy products.

A pregnant woman has cause to be concerned about potentially dangerous substances in her food. Chemicals that are carcinogenic or poisonous may also have adverse effects on the fetus. But what is her recourse? Though most women could certainly live without hot dogs and diet soda during pregnancy, they obviously cannot give up all meats, fish, and produce. Moderation in diet seems to be the most practical answer. Other recommendations:

- Eat a variety of quality foods.
- Avoid highly processed foods.
- Thoroughly wash fruits and vegetables.
- Grow your own produce.

Feeding the newborn

Another important nutritional matter that women should consider during pregnancy is how they will feed their newborn infants. The issues of breast- versus bottle-feeding have been hotly debated in recent years, as many women have decided to return to the "old way"—breast-feeding their babies. Baby feeding is, obviously, an individual decision, though many people—husband, family, friends—may try to influence the choice. Life-style after delivery is also a consideration for many women.

Some matters to think about:

• *Breast-feeding.* The American Academy of Pediatrics recently urged that every mother breast-feed her infant unless she or the baby has a specific physical condition that would make nursing impossible. The primary reason for such a statement is that human milk is uniquely suited to the metabolism of the newborn. Specifically, this means that:

• The *protein* in breast milk is more digestible and is used more efficiently than the protein in cow's milk.

• The *fats* in breast milk are better absorbed than those in cow's milk.

• Though the *iron* content of breast milk is low, it is sufficient to meet the needs of a full-term infant until its birth weight is tripled. The low iron content is actually beneficial in another respect. Two substances in breast milk, lactoferrin and transferrin, help prevent the growth of dangerous bacteria in the infant's intestinal tract. But iron in certain amounts inhibits the anti-bacterial action of these substances. The amount of iron in breast milk, however, is not high enough to make lactoferrin and transferrin ineffective.

Other health reasons for breast-feeding:

• Breast milk (and the colostrum that precedes the milk) contains important antibodies that protect the infant from infection during the first months of life.

• Breast-feeding helps speed the return of the uterus to its normal size.

• Breast-feeding avoids the danger of contamination, which may occur when formula is prepared.

On a practical level:

• Breast milk is available quickly, and at any time and in any place.

• Breast-feeding is cheaper than bottle-feeding, since there's no formula and special equipment to buy.

Finally, women who breast-feed say they experience a special feeling of closeness with their infants during nursing. This may be because breast milk is one thing *only* a mother can provide for her infant.

Is breast milk safe?

In recent years, there has been concern that breast milk contains harmful quantities of pesticide and other chemical residues. Some experts feel that the amount of these substances in breast milk can lead to illness in the infant and later susceptibility to cancer.

Chemicals get into breast milk chiefly through foods the mother eats. Meat and high-fat dairy products are particularly likely to contain pesticide residues. Lake and river fish may be tainted by dangerous substances from industrial pollution.

To reduce the dangers from pesticides and other toxic chemicals, nursing mothers should:

• Try to eat lean meats and low-fat dairy products.
• Trim excess fat from meats; skim fat from soups and stews.
• Avoid lake and river fish. Eat ocean fish.
• Avoid contact with garden pesticides.

Still, most experts think it is advisable to breast-feed, since the advantages outweigh possible problems from these contaminants.

Nutritional needs during lactation

Basically, a woman who breast-feeds should follow the same nutritional guidelines she did while pregnant. She should eat well and not try to diet. (The Daily Food Guide on page 74 indicates nutritional requirements for the lactating woman.) In addition, the nursing woman needs to drink plenty of fluids to maintain her milk supply. The prenatal vitamin and mineral supplement or regular multiple vitamin may be continued throughout lactation. In general, drugs should be avoided, as they pass to the infant through the milk. Also, oral contraceptives reduce milk supply. They should be avoided and another method of birth control should be used.

How long you breast-feed is completely up to you. Whether you nurse for a few weeks or a year or more, the baby will benefit. Pregnant women who want to know how long they might be breast-feeding (because of job commitments or family considerations) should understand that the decision to wean is flexible. Nursing need not cause an upheaval in career or family plans. Many women nurse their babies successfully while holding down jobs outside the home. Some books on breast-feeding offer new mothers detailed advice on how to combine nursing and working.

For information on breast-feeding, pregnant women can contact their local chapter of the La Leche League, or write or call the central office: La Leche League International, Inc., 9616 Minneapolis Avenue, Franklin Park, Illinois 60131. Telephone: 312-455-7730. In some areas, there may also be nutrition classes for pregnant women that will provide valuable information on breast- and bottle-feeding.

• **Bottle-feeding.** Though breast-feeding is on the upsurge, most American women still bottle-feed their infants. Certainly, today's formulas meet all of the baby's nutritional needs. In addition, many experts feel that infants fare equally well on breast or bottle, as long as they're fed with love and a sense of closeness.

Many women feel bottle-feeding fits their life-style better than breast-feeding. They find the bottle more convenient if they work outside the home or have other children to care for. Especially during the first weeks after delivery, breast-feeding mothers can feel somewhat tied down to an infant who nurses frequently. Bottle-feeding makes it possible for the mother to take a "breather" from baby feeding, and allows others, particularly the father, to spend some special time with the infant. Some mothers choose bottle-feeding because they feel they would be self-conscious about breast-feeding.

Many women bottle-feed because they prefer knowing exactly how much milk the baby is getting. Also, since formula is generally digested less quickly than breast milk, bottle-fed infants may sleep through the night sooner than breast-fed babies, and may also sleep for longer periods during the day.

Two potential problems with bottle feeding:

• Bottle-fed infants may gain more weight than they should because there is a tendency to make them *finish* a bottle instead of just drink the amount they need.

• Bottle-fed infants seem to have a harder time than breast-fed babies in going from a nipple to a cup.

Drugs

The food a pregnant woman eats can help form the fetus into a strong baby with every chance for a healthy, active future. Other substances that a pregnant woman voluntarily ingests may have the opposite effect: they may so damage the fetus that it can never enjoy a normal life. Although not all the evidence is in on all substances discussed below, abstaining or at least limiting your intake while pregnant is emphatically recommended.

Alcohol

While some people still do not consider alcohol a drug, the potential health hazards from alcohol consumption are well known. A recent addition to the list of these hazards is the danger to the fetus when its mother drinks. Alcohol passes to the fetus in the same concentration as exists in the mother's bloodstream. If a pregnant woman is drunk, the fetus will be drunk, too, but its immature system will be much less equipped to deal with the alcohol.

Fetal alcohol syndrome (FAS)

Considerable research has been done on the hazards to the fetus from alcohol. Initially, this research looked at women who were heavy drinkers. Studies showed that expectant mothers who drank six average-size drinks (about three ounces of absolute alcohol) or more a day were more likely to produce children with a variety of defects. These defects, subsequently described as the fetal alcohol syndrome (FAS), include:

- mental retardation, malformed brain, lack of coordination, hyperactivity, poor attention span
- height and weight deficiency at birth that rarely can be overcome in later life
- facial abnormalities, such as small eyes, short nose, and flat midface, and other abnormalities that have become the "trademark" of FAS children

Besides suffering from FAS, some babies born of chronic alcoholics may themselves be addicted and display the early stages of liver disease.

More startling than the correlation between heavy drinking and birth defects is new evidence that *moderate* alcohol consumption may affect fetal growth and development. Researchers at the University of Washington, Seattle, found evidence that women who drank more than one ounce of absolute alcohol a day in early pregnancy ran a risk of having babies showing some signs of FAS—though the abnormalities were less severe than those in infants of heavy drinkers.

One ounce of absolute alcohol is equivalent to about two mixed drinks (or about two beers or two glasses of wine)—an amount certainly within the definition of "social drinking." Since no studies have shown that any amount of alcohol is truly safe during pregnancy, many experts believe pregnant women should not drink at all. Some of these experts are even encouraging the government to require warning labels on liquor bottles stating that drinking during pregnancy may cause birth defects.

Nicotine

When a woman smokes during pregnancy, she deprives her baby of some vital oxygen and also changes fetal blood pressure and heart rate. But what do these changes mean to the infant? For some time, cigarette smoking during pregnancy has been linked to lower birth weight (about one-half pound less) and smaller placentas. Some researchers think that nicotine or carbon monoxide directly retards fetal growth. Others believe that because smoking affects the mother's blood circulation, the fetus may not get all the nutrients it needs from maternal blood.

Other information about smoking during pregnancy to consider:

• Miscarriage and stillbirth are thought to occur more frequently when a pregnant woman smokes.

• There is evidence that maternal smoking may increase the risk of birth defects, and also slow physical and mental development through age seven.

• A researcher at the University of Copenhagen found signs of blood-vessel damage—which may lead to hardening of the arteries or heart attack in later life—among newborns of mothers who smoked.

• Respiratory infections appear to be more prevalent in children whose mothers smoked during pregnancy.

According to an article in *Family Health* magazine, smoking *before* pregnancy increases the likelihood of placenta previa (a condition in which the placenta attaches low in the uterus, and which may lead to premature birth) and of damage to areas of the placenta that may result in fetal or perinatal death. The article also states that women who smoke *during* pregnancy are more likely to deliver prematurely; have twice the chance of developing a placental abruption (premature detachment of the placenta from the uterus, which may seriously endanger the fetus); and increase significantly the risk that their babies will suffer sudden infant death syndrome (crib death).

Caffeine

Recently, studies have been publicized that indicate that pregnant women who drink large amounts of coffee increase their chances of having a miscarriage, stillbirth, or premature or malformed infant. One study even suggests that the father's caffeine consumption may contribute to these problems.

These reports are based on animal and human research done in the United States and other countries. Not all the studies set strict controls on factors other than caffeine ingestion (such as cigarette smoking or alcohol consumption) that might account for the obstetric complications or birth defects. However, some of the research indicates that caffeine, in relatively small amounts, may act with, or increase the effects of, other agents, such as radiation, and cause fetal malformation.

Researchers disagree on how much caffeine a pregnant woman can safely consume. Some say heavy coffee drinking (more than eight cups a day) during early pregnancy is most dangerous. Others believe that women should avoid caffeine completely throughout their pregnancies. Though the evidence is not conclusive, the safest course seems to be for pregnant women to avoid drinking large amounts of coffee, tea, or cola. The nutritive value of these drinks is low, anyway, and more healthful beverages could be substituted, at least for nine months.

Marijuana

Researchers have found no hard evidence that marijuana causes malformations in human fetuses. In lab animals, high doses of marijuana have produced some deformities but are more frequently linked to fetal growth retardation and death. The risk of chromosomal damage to children whose mothers smoked marijuana when pregnant has not been substantiated.

LSD

The literature on LSD and birth defects is not conclusive. In some studies, women who used the drug seemed more likely to have babies suffering from abnormalities, including chromosomal abnormalities, than women who did not use LSD. In a few cases, malformed infants have been reported who were born to mothers who took LSD even before conception. However, other research suggests these abnormalities were due to other factors and that LSD use was incidental to the defect.

Heroin

The use of heroin during pregnancy appears to increase the chances of perinatal death, prematurity, and low birth weight. The narcotic has not yet been connected to increased fetal deformities. But heroin users risk addicting the fetus, and other health problems associated with an addict's life may further endanger fetal well-being.

Medications

As indicated previously, all medications a pregnant woman takes will reach the fetus, and some can cause fetal malformation, disease, and even death. Because thousands of children were born with deformed arms and legs, the effects of the sedative Thalidomide on the fetus have been tragically discovered. Powerful anti-cancer drugs and drugs for a hyperactive thyroid gland have also been shown to be teratogenic. Some other drugs are *suspected* of increasing the risk of birth defects or of increasing the potential for still other drugs to cause birth defects. With a large number of other medications, though, the effect on the fetus is unknown.

To be safe, then, a pregnant woman should avoid all drugs and *never self-medicate,* particularly during the first trimester, when fetal organs are developing rapidly. But at *no point* in her pregnancy should a woman take medicine without first consulting her doctor. Of course, a preexisting medical condition in the pregnant woman, such as epilepsy, heart disease, or high blood pressure, or the onset of an illness, may make medication necessary. In these cases, the need of the mother must be weighed against possible effects on the fetus.

• *Aspirin.* Over the years, different studies on animals have shown that very large doses of aspirin and related drugs, called salicylates, cause a variety of birth defects. In humans, however, the evidence is not so clear-cut. Some researchers see a correlation between regular aspirin use in the first trimester and maternal anemia, difficult and delayed labors, increased congenital malformations, and stillbirth. Taking too much aspirin toward the end of pregnancy may cause problems, too. Both maternal and fetal blood-clotting mechanisms may be upset.

• *Tranquilizers.* In 1976, the U.S. Food and Drug Administration ordered that labels be placed on some widely prescribed tranquilizers warning that the drugs may cause fetal malformations if taken during the first trimester of pregnancy. This action reflected the findings of studies that indicated women who take Valium (diazepam), Librium (chlordiazepoxide), and Miltown (meprobamate) early in pregnancy may have children with heart and nervous-system defects, and also cleft lips and palates. This tranquilizer research is not conclusive, however, and studies done with animals do not provide clear-cut answers, either. Nevertheless, it seems wise for a pregnant woman to avoid these drugs.

• *Oral contraceptives.* The correlation between oral contraceptives and birth defects is not well established. But some researchers have noticed an increased number of heart and skeletal abnormalities in infants whose mothers took oral contraceptives in the early weeks of pregnancy.

• *Diuretics.* Diuretics, especially the potent thiazide diuretics, can cause a number of undesirable side effects in the mother and can also harm the fetal blood system. Prescribing diuretics for pregnant women was more common in the past than it is today. Many physicians used to believe that diuretics were needed to counteract the edema of pregnancy and also to prevent toxemia.

• *Amphetamines.* In the past, amphetamines, which suppress appetite, were prescribed for pregnant women in order to control their weight. We've come to learn the dangers of this practice, since pregnant women must eat well. Amphetamines have also been shown to be teratogenic in some mammals. Some studies indicate that when these drugs are taken in early pregnancy they may produce a variety of malformations in humans, too. But because other reports dispute these data, the verdict on amphetamines is not yet in.

• *Antihistamines.* In lab animals, some antihistamines appear to cause birth defects such as cleft lips and palates. However, studies in humans indicate no higher incidence of fetal deformity when the mother takes these drugs. Certain antihistamines may affect the liver function of newborns when their mothers have taken the drugs during pregnancy.

Antibiotics

• *Tetracycline.* The use of tetracycline early in pregnancy involves two problems. In the fetus, this antibiotic affects the enamel and can also cause yellow or orange staining of the first set of teeth. There is also some evidence that tetracycline may retard the growth of the fetus's long bones. In the mother, large doses of tetracycline may promote serious liver damage.

• *Penicillin.* For many years, pregnant women have used penicillin with no apparent ill effects on the fetus or on themselves.

• *Erythromycin.* Often prescribed when a person is allergic to penicillin, erythromycin appears to be safe for women to take during pregnancy.

• *Sulfa drugs.* This group of drugs appears to have no teratogenic effects on either humans or lab animals. However, hyperbilirubinemia ("yellow jaundice") can be induced in infants whose mothers take sulfa drugs near delivery.

If you must have X rays

X rays are a common diagnostic tool. So common, in fact, that many women are routinely exposed to medical X rays during pregnancy—often before they know they are pregnant, and sometimes during the later months. One fairly common procedure is designed specifically for pregnant women. X-ray pelvimetry, a high-dose X-ray exam, is used to determine the size of the baby and the size of the mother's bony pelvis to see if vaginal birth is possible.

Just as we have become more aware of drugs and environmental hazards, many physicians and geneticists have become concerned about radiation. Are X rays harmful to the fetus? If so, should a pregnant woman consider abortion if she has had X rays? Should she avoid X rays even if her physician tells her they are necessary?

Because of rapid cell growth, fetuses are more susceptible than adults to radiation damage. One University of California study concluded that a fetus may be harmed by radiation at any point during pregnancy. Spontaneous abortion can occur if massive doses of X rays are administered to the mother in the early weeks of pregnancy; congenital malformations may result if X rays are done later during the first trimester; and leukemia may strike the fetus in childhood if X rays are administered during later trimesters.

But knowing that X rays can cause damage is not enough because a fetus, like an adult, can remain healthy despite the minimal exposure involved in many examinations. The question is: *How much* radiation can increase the risk of injury to the fetus? Unfortunately, no one knows the answer, although we do know what kinds of procedures deliver greater amounts of radiation to the fetus. According to Priscilla Laws, Ph.D., a professor of physics who has done research on radiation for Ralph Nader's Public Citizen Health Research Group, and who wrote *X-Rays: More Harm than*

Good?, the fetus receives the most exposure from X rays directed to the abdomen and digestive tract, kidneys, reproductive organs, urinary tract, and lower back. Nevertheless, some researchers point out that procedures for X raying even these parts of the body are safe for the fetus.

Most physicians agree that there may be some risk from X rays but that the risk is a small one. In light of this, they say that necessary X-ray procedures are acceptable during pregnancy but should be prescribed conservatively.

If you are confused about X rays, the following guidelines may help:

• If X rays have been prescribed and you think you may be pregnant, be sure to tell your physician, the radiologist, and the technician of your suspicions.

• Both the American College of Radiology and the American College of Obstetricians and Gynecologists agree that while pregnancy must be considered, medically necessary X rays should not be postponed or canceled because of the remote risk of fetal harm.

• If a physician prescribes X rays, ask whether they may be delayed until after delivery. If they are necessary without delay, be certain s/he or you check with your obstetrician or nurse-midwife before proceeding. See if you can wear lead shielding. Finally, as Professor Laws notes, never agree to an X ray to diagnose pregnancy. There are other pregnancy tests that can be performed.

• Should you choose abortion if you are unwittingly exposed to a large dose of radiation in early pregnancy? Most authorities think not. The American College of Radiology states that "interruption of pregnancy is *never* justified because of the radiation risk to the embryo/fetus from a diagnostic x-ray examination." The medical society adds that if an abortion were performed on every pregnant woman who had had an abdominal X ray, anywhere from 1,000 to 10,000 healthy fetuses would be sacrificed for the possible one fetus with abnormalities. The American College of Obstetricians and Gynecologists notes that the risk to a fetus from diagnostic radiation is substantially less than the natural incidence of birth defects.

If, however, a pregnant woman has received a dose of radiation larger than 10 rads (this would be an extraordinarily high dose; most procedures involve less than 1 rad), the risk of fetal death, congenital malformation, retardation, and even minor alterations in childhood behavior is significant. The possibility of therapeutic abortion should be discussed with your physician. S/he will take into account the amount of radiation absorbed by the fetus, and the state of fetal development, in trying to judge what effect the radiation may have had on the fetus. It should be pointed out, however, that even at 10 rads the risk of anomalies is a small one.

Sources for This Chapter

The major sources of nutrition information for this chapter were:

American College of Obstetricians and Gynecologists. *Assessment of Maternal Nutrition.* Chicago: American College of Obstetricians and Gynecologists, and American Dietetic Association, 1978.

Brewer, Gail Sforza, and Tom Brewer. *What Every Pregnant Woman Should Know: The Truth About Diet and Drugs in Pregnancy.* New York: Random House, 1977.

Carson, Mary B., ed. *The Womanly Art of Breastfeeding.* Rev. ed. Franklin Park, Ill.: La Leche League International, 1963.

Committee on Maternal Nutrition, National Research Council. *Maternal Nutrition and the Course of Pregnancy.* Washington, D.C.: National Academy of Sciences, 1970.

Davis, Adelle. *Let's Eat Right to Keep Fit.* Rev. ed. New York: Harcourt Brace Jovanovich, 1970; New American Library, 1970.

————. *Let's Have Healthy Children.* Expanded ed. New York: Harcourt Brace Jovanovich, 1972; New American Library, 1972.

Eiger, Marvin S., and Sally W. Olds. *The Complete Book of Breastfeeding.* New York: Workman Publishing Co., 1972; Bantam Books, 1973.

Lappé, Frances Moore. *Diet for a Small Planet.* Rev. ed. New York: Ballantine Books, 1975.

Maternal and Child Health Unit, California Department of Health. *Nutrition During Pregnancy and Lactation.* Sacramento: California Department of Health, 1978.

Null, Gary, and Steve Null. *Protein for Vegetarians.* New York: Pyramid Books, 1974.

Pryor, Karen. *Nursing Your Baby.* Rev. ed. New York: Harper & Row, 1973; Pocket Books, 1977.

Robinson, Corinne Hogden. *Fundamentals of Normal Nutrition.* 2d ed. New York: Macmillan, 1973.

CHAPTER SIX
The Emotional Side

In the rush to get maternity clothes, the shock of your new shape, and the sheer physicality of it all, it's easy to forget that pregnancy is as much a psychological state as it is a physical one. Whether you think of it as a hurdle to adulthood, a rounding out of your family, an unexpected joy, or simply a mistake, it is nevertheless a period of transition. Emotional sands shift until equilibrium is reached. The way you respond to your pregnancy is as important to your growth as are the other landmarks of your life.

We all come to pregnancy with certain attitudes and expectations about the process. Feelings reach back to childhood: some of us may vividly remember the excitement or anxiety surrounding the arrival of a new sibling; some of us have blotted out the memories but not the responses. Twenty-four-year-old Marcia, herself the older of two daughters, noticed these feelings very soon after the birth of her first child. "When Jessica was born, I had an amazing sensation. I thought that she looked exactly like my younger sister, and it wasn't until several weeks later that I could shake that feeling." In some ways, she was recalling the birth of her sister; it may even have been that some of her attitudes toward her daughter were remnants from the past, too.

A sense of the future

Other emotions result from the almost intense planning for the future, as we begin to imagine how our children will enrich or intrude upon our later lives. During the many months of pregnancy we begin to develop a range of feelings unique to the experience. All of us imagine what our child will look like; to make it more real, we may even fantasize about whether the baby will grow to be musical or athletic, whether it will be intellectual or artistic, whether it will be sensitive, funny, or sweet. One mother of a three-year-old laughed as she said, "When I was pregnant I imagined Joey to be all the things that I wished *I* were. It turned out that Joey was unlike anything I could imagine." There's nothing wrong with the daydreams we have during pregnancy; psychologists tell us that it's healthy to personify the infant within us.

Emotional states are often tied to *physical* changes during pregnancy. Such discomforts as fatigue, nausea, backache, or excessive weight gain can make us feel depressed or unsure about our pregnancies. On the positive side, not worrying about getting pregnant can help make sex more spontaneous and creative. Even a cleared-up complexion—the result of prenatal hormone activity—might help us feel better about our "condition."

Actually, increased hormone production may *cause* mood swings: some pregnant women feel exhilarated one moment, close to tears the next. It's important to realize that the enormous changes our bodies undergo during pregnancy make all these emotions normal, and that these changes of mood also help pave the way for a good adjustment later.

Many factors influence the way we feel

How we (and our partners) feel about our pregnancy can be influenced by more than just physical changes. Other factors that may affect our emotional outlook on pregnancy include:

• *Timing.* Was the pregnancy an accident or was it expected? Even if we want children, an unplanned pregnancy can be a shock. And if we're unsure about parenthood, it may be seriously upsetting and sufficient reason to seek professional counseling. On the other hand, getting pregnant unexpectedly has proved a joyful surprise for many couples. If we've been trying a long time to conceive, we may have a hard time believing it's finally happened.

Women who have suffered miscarriages may view even a wanted pregnancy with apprehension. "When I conceived again, after three miscarriages, I tried to ignore my pregnancy," said one college teacher. "I guess I had invested so much before, I couldn't face losing it all again. It wasn't until my fifth month that I felt joy again."

Marital status. The state of our marriage or whether we are married can have a significant effect when we step into still another life role. Pregnancy generally enhances a good marital relationship. Occasionally it will even stabilize a shaky one, but more often the new concerns and stresses that arise during pregnancy further damage the already deteriorating relationship.

First or subsequent pregnancy. "For my first pregnancy, I felt like Lady Madonna. With my second, I just wanted to get through it," noted a mother of two preschool boys. A sense of wonder and excitement usually touches every aspect of a first pregnancy. Every twinge, every ache, is new and special. For some women this holds true even in their eighth pregnancy. For many women, however, subsequent pregnancies lose some of the novelty of the first.

The demands of another child can also affect how we enjoy a pregnancy. If we can't find time to rest or must be extremely attentive to another's needs, we may find ourselves without time for our own needs. Spacing can play a part, too. The physical strain of very close pregnancies can cause attendant psychological strain. On the other hand, some women with many years between pregnancies may doubt they'll be able to return to the "baby routine."

Career plans. If a woman has a specific career or plans for one, she may wonder if the pregnancy can be successfully integrated with her goals. Most women feel very good, some even better than usual, during pregnancy, and they continue their work or schooling right up to the time they deliver. Other women may assume that pregnancy and childbirth will not interfere with their plans, then later are disappointed or resentful if they do.

It helps to be flexible about future plans, at least until your child is several months old and you can make decisions about your career in a less emotionally charged state. One successful woman lawyer said, "When I was pregnant, I was positively compulsive about my future; at every spare minute I worried about how I would juggle my baby and my job. As it turned out, things kind of fell into place after Miranda was born. I got a housekeeper who had just stopped working for a good friend, and I was offered part-time work, even though I hadn't really been looking."

The reactions of others. When parents, friends, colleagues, and especially our husband or partner delight in our pregnancy, it naturally enhances our own joy. "My mother remembered the thrill of finding out she was pregnant. She was excited for me to have that same thrill," said one expectant mother. Hearing "You look terrific pregnant" or "We're so excited for you" can certainly help us feel good about our pregnant selves. On the other hand, lack of support, especially from people we feel close to, can be demoralizing during this important time in our lives. One woman, whose co-workers were all young and childless, remembers fielding the constant question: "Did you *want* it?" "Although I wanted my baby very much, I began to wonder if maybe I *did* make a mistake," she said.

Getting the news

Sometimes, long before a pregnancy begins, women speculate about how they'll feel during that time. Some of us may see maternity clothes and imagine how we'll look in them, or see babies and fantasize how we will act as mothers. When we actually learn we are pregnant, these feelings may surface again, along with others that might be quite different from those we anticipated.

Even if they have suspected pregnancy, many expectant couples are overjoyed and amazed when the news is confirmed. "I wanted to shout, to yell the good news in our car when Ken picked me up from the doctor's," said one woman about learning she was pregnant for the first time. Couples may feel pride at creating a new life, or be excited to take such an important life step, as so many have done before them. One father-to-be noted, "It was like I had joined the human race, when we learned Jan was pregnant."

We may be enormously curious about impending changes; we may feel happy to give our parents grandchildren. Indeed, one of the most pleasant aspects of pregnancy can be the exciting moment when you tell others the news. You may even mentally rehearse which words you'll use. Some couples view the news of a pregnancy as an affirmation or fulfillment of their marriage or sexuality. If a woman hasn't known the reason she's been feeling ill or fatigued, a confirmation of pregnancy can be a relief.

There are worries, too

The reality of pregnancy can provoke some concerns, too. After the initial rush of enthusiasm, couples may begin to wonder how the pregnancy, and eventually the baby, will affect their marriage, finances, sex lives, careers. One husband said he was afraid to have sex during his wife's entire pregnancy. "Intellectually, I knew it was all right, but I couldn't get rid of the feeling that I might hurt the baby." The resulting tension between him and his wife didn't ease until months after the birth.

Both men and women can feel trapped or overwhelmed by the commitment pregnancy signifies. Some may consider having an abortion. We may feel guilty because society tells us how happy we should be and we can't totally rid ourselves of anxiety. Also, if a woman hasn't been feeling well, negative emotions about pregnancy may be amplified. Couples and individuals may feel better, or understand their feelings better, if they can talk out their fears, either with a professional or in groups.

During pregnancy

The nine months of pregnancy provide us with time to think about the physical changes occurring in our bodies and about the baby who will change how we look at ourselves, our spouses, our careers, our futures. Feelings fluctuate during these months. The depression that may accompany weeks of nausea usually fades as the second trimester begins. The enervation of the ninth month turns to excitement as the due date approaches. Again, it's sometimes helpful to remember that many of these negative feelings are beyond our control, and that if we have a bad day, it's just a temporary condition. The emotions we have during pregnancy may be focused in certain areas:

• *Self-image.* During pregnancy, how we think about ourselves usually begins to change. Aspects of our personality, like marriage or career, are shifted to prepare for parenthood. We see ourselves with new responsibilities. We begin the transition from being self-oriented to being ready to provide the complete care our newborns demand. If the pregnancy is going well, we may feel more confident that we can accept our new role capably. But even during the easiest pregnancy, it's natural for men and women to wonder how they will function as parents. And when the pregnancy has been particularly stressful or complicated by illness, the wondering may give way to serious doubts about our abilities.

• *Preparing for the baby.* Our change in self-image may manifest itself in how we actually change our life-style. Maternity clothes are the first outward indication that a woman is pregnant. Most of us are excited when we wear them for the first time. Some women rush to buy maternity clothes before they're necessary because of the novelty. Other expectant mothers delay maternity clothes awhile, not quite believing the pregnancy is real, or fearing that they may "jinx" it, or being unready to affirm their condition to themselves or the people around them. One mother explained how she surreptitiously toured maternity shops for two months, eyeing the clothes but never buying, until finally she got up the courage to go in and make a purchase. "I *knew* I was pregnant, but couldn't really face it. The day I bought my first top was a real milestone."

Buying a layette or baby furniture also indicates acceptance of the baby. Some parents-to-be get a crib, clothes, and toilet articles together toward the end of pregnancy so they'll be set when the baby arrives. Other couples wouldn't dream of acquiring baby things until after birth. Still other expectant parents buy furniture and clothing throughout the pregnancy—maybe starting soon after the condition is confirmed.

• *Changing our surroundings.* During pregnancy we also look at our surroundings differently, as we imagine how they'll adapt to a child. Pregnancy may be the time when we make a move from an apartment to a house, to a larger apartment, or from a couples-oriented locale to a neighborhood filled with children. Without actually moving we might also see the need to change a particular room for the coming baby. So we buy paint, choose wallpaper, sew curtains, and transform the den into a nursery. Some couples find it exciting to change their environment. Others may resent the time and energy they have to expend for someone who is not actually here yet.

• *Career concerns.* Pregnancy may start both men and women thinking about their work and how it fits into their lives. A working woman's life can be particularly affected by pregnancy. But an expectant father might wonder if his job can support a family. Men who may have previously felt absolutely secure at their jobs now begin to worry about getting fired. "It was crazy. I was so wrapped up in my job—for the baby's sake—that I walked around with a knot in my stomach for nine months," said a father of two, of his experiences during his wife's first pregnancy.

Some men think about changing to jobs that pay more or have different hours. Some take on another job. Depending on how satisfying the original job was, or how much pressure is involved in having two jobs, these changes can be frustrating and stressful. An expectant mother hoping for an increase in attention and love from her partner may be upset to find the opposite to be true.

• *You and your partner.* Before you became expectant parents, you were lovers. Presumably your relationship was so fulfilling that you deliberately chose to enhance it by having a baby. Yet even strong feelings of love, affection, and closeness can be strained by the physical and emotional stresses of pregnancy. Not only do you and your partner change as individuals, but pregnancy affects the way you look at your life together.

Couples report stormy and calm times, periods of tremendous tenderness, and also, occasionally, feelings of alienation from one another. Some feelings of dissatisfaction can be traced to altered patterns of need—one partner may feel that s/he is giving more than s/he is getting. For example, an expectant father called on to perform many more household chores may feel resentful (as would an expectant mother). Although the father may not mind giving the extra *physical* support to his partner, he may have additional needs for *emotional* support that go unfulfilled.

Most women want their partners to take an active interest in their pregnancies. We're eager to share the joy of this important phase in our lives and want to be supported in the choices we make concerning it. We would like our partners to know all we are experiencing in our bodies and understand when we are physically uncomfortable.

Some women want or expect to be pampered during pregnancy, feeling this is a special, short-lived time. Sometimes we may get angry when our mate doesn't share our enthusiasm about the baby's kicks or won't commiserate about morning sickness.

Expectant fathers may need pampering, too. Though not physically affected, fathers-to-be may feel a number of emotional strains relating to pregnancy and may be unable to articulate them clearly. They may be very unsure about what pregnancy will mean for them. They may feel left out of all the attention usually showered on the mother. Sharing the pregnancy as much as possible—by taking classes, reading books, seeing the doctor or nurse-midwife together—can help eliminate misunderstandings that often arise during this time. Being particularly considerate of each other's feelings can be helpful, too.

Pregnancy can easily affect how we relate to our partners sexually. This is especially true if a physician or other expert tells us to avoid sex for any time during the pregnancy. Some women experience no change in their sexual relations during pregnancy. Others feel sex is better when birth control is unnecessary, or changing body contours make relations more exciting, or the sheer joy of the pregnancy increases desire. "My husband loved the fact that my breasts got bigger during pregnancy. He thought I was the sexiest woman in the world," said one woman.

For other couples, such physical problems as nausea or fatigue, especially in the early months, can inhibit desire or performance. Also, the fear of miscarriage or hurting the baby through sex is an anxiety many of us experience while pregnant, even though we may intellectually understand that sex will not be harmful.

Some women want sex more in early pregnancy but lose interest closer to term as they become heavier or feel ungainly. Some of us may have trouble meshing the ideas of "mother" and "sex partner" so that we can thoroughly enjoy sex during pregnancy. Some men cannot fully appreciate the physical or emotional discomforts of pregnancy that may affect their partner's sexual desires. These men feel frustrated, often, and ignored if their partner's desires do not match their own. Similarly, a woman who finds pregnancy increases her desire for sex may feel frustrated if her mate's desires are not as strong, or if he is reluctant to have sex for fear of harming the baby.

To accommodate the changes in a woman's body during pregnancy, sexual preferences may change, too. Some women find the male-superior position too uncomfortable, especially in later pregnancy. Men often feel the same about the female-superior position. Many couples prefer intercourse on their sides, from behind, or in other positions where the woman's abdomen is not in the way. When genital intercourse is not comfortable physically or psychologically—for fear of harming or disturbing the baby—we may concentrate on other forms of sexual expression such as oral sex (safe as long as air is not blown into the vagina) or mutual masturbation. Some couples find it helpful to redefine what sex means to them and see massage and "snuggling" as important sexual communication. This redefinition may remove some of the pressure to perform many of us feel at this time.

If this is a first pregnancy, you and your partner may experience strong feelings of isolation if you are not near family, or if you are the first among your friends to be expecting. Isolation can increase any anxieties parents-to-be might suffer about their baby, their relationship, and their individual identities.

Tapping into outside support systems, or developing some of their own, can be important to a couple if pregnancy seems to be creating unbridgeable gulfs between them. Any group that encourages partners to discuss the pregnancy together can be valuable— childbirth-education classes, baby-care classes, and rap groups are possibilities. Visiting the obstetrician as a couple—with both of you present in the examining room—is often a good idea. And if the people with whom you socialize are, or have recently been, expectant parents, the shared experiences can be a real boost.

Supporting each other can be continuous, hard work. For many reasons, it may be difficult to communicate with the person with whom you are closest; you may find you are reluctant to share expectations and fantasies for fear of disappointing yourself or your partner. Other couples grow *so* dependent on each other during pregnancy that breathing space is needed by both to reassert individual strengths.

Being alert to your partner's feelings and your own contributes to the continuous fine tuning necessary during pregnancy. Setting aside time together as a couple (particularly if you have other children who demand your attention) is an urgent need; setting aside time for yourself is just as important. Consider that your partner may need time alone, too.

Support can be verbal, sexual, physical, and emotional; it can mean involvement or even withdrawal. Experiment with the kinds of support that seem most appropriate to your relationship, recognizing that both partners may need to make sacrifices and concessions for later rewards. Flexibility, a sense of humor, and a willingness to share mark the parameters of a mutually supportive relationship.

• *Stress.* At times we all experience stress when we are confronted by unfamiliar or unpleasant situations. Stress may appear as a state of vague unease, or you may be badly disturbed. Your concentration, your ability to cope, and even your self-awareness dwindle when you are under stress. Throughout our lives, we develop methods of dealing with stress, and we instinctively call them up to minimize the strains that threaten us.

During pregnancy, when so many emotional and physical changes demand your energy, you may be very susceptible to stress—in your relationships, on the job, and concerning your pregnancy. You may find the old mechanisms for recovering balance no longer work. What you could manage before seems, at times, overwhelming now. Stresses may be magnified and so may their effects on the pregnant woman; the effects of stress on the fetus are unclear, although some researchers hypothesize a link between stress during pregnancy and irritability, colic, and even emotional upset in the newborn.

Some different kinds of stress you may encounter during pregnancy:

• *Built-in stresses.* These are intrinsic to your condition and are felt by nearly every pregnant woman at some point or other. These include worries about your baby's health and about labor and delivery; pressures to perform in a certain way because of, or despite, your pregnancy; concerns about how your baby will affect your marriage, career, and living arrangements; even anxiety about having weight and blood pressure measured.

• *Chronic stresses.* Pregnancy offers no special immunity to these. A high-pressure job, a shaky marriage, or a difficult child can cause a state of anxiety or even ill health that may linger for months.

• *Sudden stresses.* Again, pregnancy does not exempt you from the bone-jarring stresses we all encounter sporadically: the death of a loved one; a move away from a familiar environment; the loss of your own or your spouse's livelihood.

Though some of the causes of stress are well known, most experts aren't sure exactly how stress affects the body. Some theorize that dozens of illnesses are stress-related; others link stress to gastric disorders, heart disease, hypertension, migraine headaches, insomnia, and menstrual problems. Women under stress may also have difficulty conceiving. If you are pregnant, stress may worsen nausea or other digestive problems, bring on premature labor, make labor more difficult to cope with, and transform fleeting postpartum "blues" into a lingering depression.

Like everyone else, pregnant women are apt to overeat, drink too much, and smoke when they're under pressure. Some women may even turn to tranquilizers and other drugs to cope with daily strains. However, these outlets are particularly dangerous to the health of the mother and fetus. If you've been accustomed to relying on these methods to reduce stress, pregnancy is the time to learn different approaches.

You *can* diminish stress. You can, during pregnancy, develop new ways of coping that can be used not only for these nine months but beyond:

• Communicate your worries to someone you trust. If you're apprehensive about birth, speak with women who have recently experienced it. If your partner seems distant and you feel pressure about your relationship, try to air the problem.

• Learn to recognize the symptoms of stress. Some of these might be listlessness, depression, inability to relax, changing sleep patterns, withdrawal from family and friends.

• Educate yourself about your physiology, about your job rights, about insurance, about anything that concerns you. Take the offensive and meet worries head-on.

• Sit and think things through calmly. Organize your daily tasks. If your job involves a lot of responsibility, you may be particularly subject to stresses during pregnancy, when fatigue, irritability, and distraction may be more common. (Recent studies have shown that women in middle management are especially susceptible to stress.) If you can set up daily plans and schedules for projects, if you can set goals and analyze how to meet them, you can avoid being overwhelmed by less essential tasks.

• Be sure you have adequate time and privacy for yourself each day. If you don't, you may feel pulled in all directions at once and resentful about not being able to enjoy the pregnancy or think about your baby.

• Stress for one person may be a mere annoyance to another. Take a cue from your more easygoing friends in dealing with some of your stresses.

• Try physical release. Walking, yoga, and even simple stretching are all helpful when your body is tense and tired.

• Give yourself a "free day" periodically. No visitors, no phone calls, no interruptions. Read, swim, bathe, walk, or just stay in bed if it seems that's what will help you relax. All of us need to "recess to reassess."

• There's no way to prepare for sudden stress. Depression, lethargy, or hopelessness may engulf you; these feelings may even be healthy responses—at least for a time. If, however, you can't pull out of a tailspin, seek professional help.

• Now is the time to arrange for all the help you can afford. Hire baby-sitters, housekeepers, and cleaning services to relieve the burden of everyday chores.

•*Fears and fantasies.* With most important life changes, people experience some fears along with the excitement of change. During pregnancy, many of these fears center on our health and that of the baby. We may worry that we won't have the energy to meet the demands of our daily routine and the demands of the pregnancy. We may wonder what labor and delivery will feel like and if they will be good experiences.

Almost every pregnant woman has some fleeting fear about miscarriage or the health of her child. We wonder if the baby will be normal and if we'll be able to cope if s/he isn't. "My mother never carried to term, so I was terribly worried that my baby would be premature," said one woman. We may think about death in terms of our new responsibilities as parents. Maybe we decide to get more insurance, or think about making a will.

In a first pregnancy, it may even be difficult to pinpoint our anxiety—what we fear is the unknown. As one thirty-year-old mother of two noted, "When I was pregnant for the first time, I didn't know what was happening to my body—every ache and pain worried me." In a second or subsequent pregnancy, couples may be acutely aware of what it means to have a child, and of how dependent infants are on their parents. Second-time expectant mothers with a healthy child may fear they will not be as lucky again. We may also be concerned about how the second child will affect the first and how we'll handle the interaction. Expectant fathers may fear for the mother's health during pregnancy and childbirth.

•*Imaginings.* First-time expectant parents may have trouble imagining the changes a child will bring to their lives. We may spend some time worrying about the coming baby, but we can also have a good deal of *fun* "creating" our future child when we think about its eye and hair color, how it will look as a toddler, which parent it will look like, and will "it" be twins? We probably envision a perfect child, without tantrums, soiled diapers, or illness.

• *Parents and in-laws.* To some degree, how we feel about our pregnancy depends on how others view it. Most women want and expect support from their husbands during pregnancy and may be upset or worried when this support is not available. But the reactions of others in our families, especially parents—who are so intimately tied to our ideas of parenting—can affect our emotions. Many women find they become closer to their mothers during pregnancy. Usually we are happy to make them grandmothers. But in addition we may enjoy sharing our joys, fears, and questions with a woman who is so close to us and who has been through this experience before. Sometimes, because of the pregnancy, we feel more like adults when we deal with our mothers, or believe we understand her feelings and actions better. A supportive mother who welcomes our pregnancy can make us feel more positive about the experience and eager to have our own child. Talking with our mothers during pregnancy may evoke memories of our own childhood. We may evaluate how we were raised and imagine how we'll mother our own children.

Some women say they feel a sense of rivalry with their mothers over their choice of birth methods, home birth or anesthesia. Our mothers may wonder why we are choosing to breast-feed, for example, when bottles worked perfectly well for them. Our mothers might feel that implicit in these choices about pregnancy and childbirth is a criticism of how they handled the experiences.

Some mothers take over during a daughter's pregnancy—suggesting which doctor or hospital to choose,' which maternity clothes or crib to buy. One soon-to-be-grandmother, aghast that her daughter had chosen a young suburban obstetrician, convinced her daughter to switch to an old family friend—who was twice as expensive, farther away, and not very open to questions. The angry daughter switched back, unwilling to listen to any other suggestions. In this way, we may come to resent our mothers' interference. As adults, during such an important time in our lives, we feel strongly about making our own decisions.

We may experience many of the same feelings with our mothers-in-law, depending on the closeness of the relationship. Yet we may be less bothered by suggestions from an in-law, simply because they don't carry the same emotional weight as they would if they came from our own mothers. A supportive mother-in-law can be helpful, although it can be more difficult to be honest with our in-laws if we feel they are intruding on our decisions about pregnancy and childbirth. Expectant fathers may welcome the support our mothers or their own mothers offer because it relieves some of the pressure *they* may feel to be constantly understanding of our needs. But they can also feel a bit left out of the close female relationships, or resent the interference.

During pregnancy, the expectant father may also look back to his childhood and wonder how he will function as a father. He may feel strongly that the pregnancy ties him more closely to his own father, and thus may experience many of the same feelings mothers and daughters do. Some men feel they have proved themselves to their parents or in-laws by fathering a child. But they may also feel resentment if their role as a family provider is being severely scrutinized by these same people. A sharing, positive father can be helpful and reassuring for a father-to-be, who may not completely realize what lies ahead for him.

• *The extended family.* Sometimes married couples live with the husband's or wife's parents. Whether or not this situation is temporary, it can affect the way a couple accepts a pregnancy and their future child, and how they feel about themselves as parents. It's true that parents who live with you can share the responsibilities of running a household. On the other hand, during pregnancy you may have an especially strong need for privacy. Inevitably, there will be tension, because this is a time of change and of restructured relationships. Living with your parents may tend to reinforce your image of yourself as a child, when, in fact, you would prefer to see yourself as an adult. But if you can arrange for enough privacy and be candid about your needs, you may find benefits in an extended-family environment.

• *Your other children and sibling rivalry.* The prospect of a new baby in the family can cause an upheaval in a child's world, no matter how old s/he is. When told a baby's coming, the older child may be excited, fascinated, and proud that, like many neighborhood friends, s/he will have a sibling, too. On the other hand, the child may worry about his mother's changing shape, resent having to move to a different bedroom, or puzzle about mommy's sudden lack of energy. A child may be particularly anxious if s/he sees Mother vomiting, or in some way thinks that she may be ill.

A pre-verbal child may also take note of the mother's condition, even though s/he doesn't understand what pregnancy means. If mommy is irritable or slower to respond to a toddler's needs, the child may be bewildered or even upset, and may turn to the father more frequently. Toddlers may not know what a baby will mean, but they certainly know something is different.

You can help make your child's experience with a new baby a positive one by trying to prepare her/him during your pregnancy. Let your child's questions guide your explanation of pregnancy and birth. Simple answers are the best way to begin. If your child wants to know more, s/he will probably keep probing. If you sense your child is disturbed about your pregnancy and unable to communicate fears, try to draw him out tactfully. Don't force responses. If your child doesn't want to feel the baby kicking or help set up the crib, don't pressure. When your child expresses an interest, appropriate books, movies, toys, and often just seeing other babies can be beneficial.

Your child may not exhibit many emotional difficulties during your pregnancy. But your departure for the hospital and the subsequent separation from you may be extremely upsetting. Again, preparation is vital. Depending on the child's age, you may be able to explain matter-of-factly that you'll soon be going to the hospital to have the baby; that Grandma or Mrs. Peters will be coming to take care of her/him; and that when you come home you'll be bringing the new baby with you. When you're in the hospital, take advantage of sibling visitation programs, if available, to allay some of your child's anxiety about separation.

CHAPTER SEVEN
Methods of Giving Birth

"Are you going to have natural childbirth?" This may be one of the questions most often asked of an expectant couple, but it can be the most difficult to answer. Even if you are taking a preparation course with the aim of having a nonmedicated labor and birth, it's hard to know, particularly if this is your first baby, what labor and birth will feel like, how you will respond to contractions, whether you will want medication for pain relief. If you *should* need something "to take the edge off," if you are given, for example, an epidural anesthetic, or if your physician injects a local anesthetic to suture an episiotomy, have you had *natural* childbirth? What does "natural" mean, anyway?

Natural, as it turns out, doesn't mean very much. Certainly not when it is applied to the various methods that teach parents to deal—nonmedically—with the discomforts of labor. In the first place, it doesn't seem *natural* to take a course in childbirth. Didn't our ancestors—even some of our grandmothers—give birth armed only with memories of other births and accompanied by the supporting hands of their women friends and attendants? There is nothing natural about breathing patterns and techniques that take weeks to learn, about muscle conditioning or controlled relaxation of the body—all vital components of any "natural"-childbirth course. And it's not natural to change one's whole outlook and understanding of birth. Yet this is precisely what many natural-childbirth instructors teach.

Preparing for birth

It's easier to understand the goals of today's childbirth educators if we toss out the vague ideal of natural childbirth and replace it with the concept of *prepared* childbirth, of undertaking a whole conditioning program—physical, mental, and in some cases spiritual—for childbirth.

Many more of us need prepared childbirth than need natural—that is, uneducated—childbirth. Dr. Grantly Dick-Read, a pioneer in the unmedicated birth movement, pointed out decades ago the anxieties many women bring to childbirth. These anxieties are not difficult to understand, especially for women today. Few of us have ever seen a human birth or stayed beside a laboring woman. Snatches of conversations about labor don't build a complete picture, and fragments of knowledge don't give us the confidence to face our own birth experiences. How many of us can even claim to understand the physiology of birth?

Even how we order our priorities affects our birth experiences. Because so many of us pursue a career before we create children, we devote much more of our energy and thoughts to jobs than to future pregnancies and infants. Until we become pregnant we may not be interested in hearing of or learning about our friends' birth experiences. Indeed, with our friends as busy as we, it may be that everyone we know is childless. Add to these obstacles the fantasies about birth that gripped us as children and are now firmly rooted in our subconscious. Add also the cultural myths about birth, the excess psychological baggage we all carry, and it's understandable how ignorant and fearful so many of us can be about childbirth.

Dr. Dick-Read saw that ignorance and misinformation led to fear about birth in his patients, that fear caused tension, and that tension contributed to the degree of pain experienced by laboring women. He correctly saw the need to prepare his patients for the experience of birth. While many educators have through the years adapted his methods or developed new ones, no one has disputed the need for preparation. Comfortable childbirth does *not* come naturally.

Although most of us have heard of the Lamaze—also called the psychoprophylactic—method of pain relief, there are many other methods. Some childbirth educators incorporate a variety of philosophies and techniques in their courses, and others focus on a specific area, such as home birth or breast-feeding or child care, but include birthing techniques.

What birth classes teach

Birth classes may have different philosophical and psychological orientations, too. In some, mothers are taught to separate themselves from the birthing process; in others, mothers learn to harmonize with the forces at work in their bodies. Some teachers place great emphasis on the family; others focus on the emotional growth experienced by the birthing mother. Discussing your goals and interests with a childbirth instructor before you sign up for a course can be extremely helpful. All birth classes, however, include these basics:

• *Education about birth.* You will learn about the structure and function of the sex organs, about the physiology of pregnancy, labor, and delivery, and sometimes about breast-feeding. When a woman is armed with such knowledge, the unique sensations experienced during labor and birth can be anticipated and consequently are less likely to be feared.

• *Relaxation techniques.* One of the crucial skills a woman needs during labor, to dispel what Dick-Read called the "fear-tension-pain syndrome," is the ability to relax. This does not mean the ability to sleep, but rather the ability to release tension in the muscles. (If you have studied yoga, you can appreciate the distinction.) Surprisingly, this is a skill that must be learned well before labor begins, so that it can be put into use almost automatically during even the most intense contractions. All childbirth-education courses recognize relaxation as an effective way of minimizing pain.

• *Breathing techniques.* We breathe differently in different situations. For example, when we're nervous, we tend to take shallow, irregular breaths; when we're relaxed, deeper, slower breaths. Childbirth educators teach different breathing patterns for each stage of labor. Some say the breathing techniques have *physiological* value because correct breathing lifts the abdomen—or the diaphragm (depending on the technique)—off the uterus. Correct breathing also prevents hyperventilation and encourages relaxation. Other birthing methods hold that their breathing techniques simply focus the laboring woman's attention away from contractions.

• *Exercises.* If you can use your body correctly, certain discomforts of pregnancy can be minimized. Later, physical conditioning can be of great help during the hard work of labor. It's not surprising, then, that exercises are taught in all childbirth-preparation classes. The exercises do not differ that much from one method to another. Besides conditioning you for pregnancy and birth, the exercises promote relaxation and correct breathing.

• **_The partner's role._** Practically all classes encourage the father (or someone close to and supportive of the mother) to be present and "coaching" during labor and birth. His activities may include help with breathing and relaxation patterns, massage, and communication with hospital personnel for the mother. The father's, or partner's, contribution is seen as essential to a comfortable birth, not only for the mechanical aid he can provide but also for his calm, stabilizing influence, which can really help a mother gain control over the course of her labor.

Can it really be painless?

Childbirth educators in the United States rarely tell parents that they can achieve a "painless" birth, even though that was the goal Dr. Lamaze envisioned. Whether it is culturally or physically generated, most of us do feel greater or lesser degrees of discomfort through labor, and pain during the forty-five minutes or so of transition. While preparing for birth can help immensely, most women should understand that labor probably will not be completely painless.

It is precisely the idea of pain, however, that causes some grumbling in the women's movement. Why not, some say, take full advantage of the anesthetics and analgesics we are offered? Are the teachings of prepared-childbirth instructors antiwoman because they urge us to accept pain during childbirth?

Those ideas aren't new, but even with the anesthetics we have today, which are safer for mother and child than those used in childbirth decades ago when the idea of "liberation" arrived, eradicating all pain with medication is not always best for the baby or the mother.

Childbirth with minimal or no medicated relief is: (1) _safer for the baby_ because unmedicated babies are less likely to suffer depressed respiration at birth; (2) _safer for the mother_ because all anesthetics carry possible risks to the patient; and (3) _healthier for the baby_ because s/he is born alert, able to nurse, and, generally speaking, better able to respond to parents and environment.

A recent study of five hundred Lamaze-trained women in Evanston, Illinois, showed that they had fewer problems in childbirth than unprepared women in a control group matched for age, race, education, and number of previous children. The trained mothers had one-fourth as many cesarean births, and one-third the number of postdelivery infections. The babies of trained mothers had one-fifth the incidence of fetal distress.

The teachers

• *Grantly Dick-Read.* Dick-Read observed several decades ago that some women experienced pain during childbirth and others didn't. He speculated that the difference lay in preparedness. Those who were comfortable and familiar with childbirth felt less pain than those who feared it. Those who could accept it as a natural occurrence seemed more comfortable than those who resisted it. The answer, he believed, was for women to accept the childbirth process calmly. They would do so, he reasoned, only by being thoroughly educated in the mechanics of childbirth and trained in relaxation techniques. Dick-Read's deeply spiritual approach to motherhood and birth may seem foreign to some women. His philosophy may strike some as too passive a program for such a major physical event. To others, his compassionate words and deep respect for the laboring woman are highly welcome. Following his method, exercises and breathing techniques are taught—although not usually in so structured a program as that offered in the Lamaze program. The Dick-Read method also provides instruction in the physiology of labor and delivery.

• *Fernand Lamaze.* Lamaze's concept, based on research conducted in the Soviet Union, was to *condition* women for labor. He sought to teach women to respond to contractions with specific sets of breathing patterns. The laboring woman would be so intent on carrying out these patterns correctly that her attention would be focused away from the pain of contractions. He developed specific breathing patterns for each stage of labor. In addition, muscle relaxation was taught as an automatic response to uterine activity.

Body-building exercises, education about birth, and a clearly defined role for the father are also part of today's Lamaze program, which usually consists of six classes taken during the last trimester. Compared with Dick-Read's approach, the Lamaze method is highly structured. Many couples, especially first-time parents, are happy to receive detailed instructions about what to do during labor. Some critics, however, say that the Lamaze method tends to disassociate the mother from the birth experience and to deprive her of an awesome psychological and sensual experience, because instead of participating in it, she is working to ignore it. Of course, there can be a sensuality and participation in the breathing and relaxing rhythms that are established in harmony with your contractions. And the emphasis some instructors place on the father's spiritual growth can make birth a deeply shared experience.

• *Sheila Kitzinger.* Kitzinger originated the psychosexual approach, which stresses the sexual and psychological aspects of birth. Kitzinger sees pregnancy and birth as emotional milestones and the physical sensations of birth as intensely satisfying and thrilling. To her, anesthetics rob women of those feelings.

Kitzinger formulated a philosophy and method that make all trained mothers enthusiastic participants. Touch relaxation, based on the woman's responsiveness to her husband's touch during labor, is a cornerstone of the Kitzinger method. Kitzinger shares with most other childbirth educators the thinking that the ability to relax muscles of the body is crucial to a comfortable childbirth. Breathing patterns are not rigid; although Kitzinger offers some excellent suggestions, the stress is on harmonizing breathing with uterine contractions. Finally, relaxation exercises, physical conditioning exercises, and education about the mechanics and emotions of birth round out the teachings.

• *Dr. Robert A. Bradley.* Bradley developed husband-coached childbirth, a method based on Dick-Read's approach but supplemented by a strong emphasis on the father's role during birth. Bradley found that for the nonanesthetized mother to achieve serenity at birth—crucial to an optimal experience—the presence of the father is essential. Weekly classes run from the sixth month until birth. Prenatal exercise programs, nutrition, relaxation techniques, and breathing patterns are taught, all involving the active participation of the partner. There is a heavy emphasis on rejection of all medication during labor and delivery.

• *Margaret Gamper.* Gamper is a registered nurse and childbirth educator in Chicago who has been teaching pregnant women for more than thirty years. Instructors in her method teach classes that women usually join in the fourth month of pregnancy and attend every other week until the eighth. Gamper classes are based on Dick-Read's theories but also include procedures developed by Gamper that include a simple approach to relaxation. A complete discussion of the physiology and psychology of labor and birth is part of the course, although some women may be uncomfortable with the stress on femininity and the very traditional approach to the male-female relationship. Abdominal breathing is taught in several variations, corresponding to the various stages of labor. (It is still a subject of debate whether abdominal or chest breathing is preferable during labor.)

Where to take classes

Classes in prepared childbirth are offered all over the country in hospitals, adult-education programs at colleges, churches and synagogues, YMCAs, community centers, teachers' homes. If you are interested in signing up for one, ask your physician for a list of teachers in your area, or contact the obstetrics department of your local hospital and speak with the head nurse.

Sign up early! Even if a class doesn't start until the seventh month of pregnancy, it may fill up as soon as it is offered. Don't expect your physician's office to enroll you in any childbirth-preparation or child-care class. This is your responsibility.

To get more information on prepared-childbirth methods and local classes, or on other issues of childbirth, these organizations can help:

International Childbirth
Education Association
P.O. Box 20852
Milwaukee, WI 53220

National Association of
Parents and Professionals
for Safe Alternatives
in Childbirth (NAPSAC)
P.O. Box 267
Marble Hill, MO 63764

Institute for Childbirth
and Family Research
2522 Dana Street
Suite 201
Berkeley, CA 94704

American Society for Psychoprophylaxis in Obstetrics
(Lamaze method)
1411 K Street N.W.
Washington, D.C. 20005

Margaret Gamper, R.N.
Executive Director
Midwest Parentcraft Center
627 Beaver Road
Glenview, IL 60625

American Academy of
Husband-Coached Childbirth
(Bradley method)
P.O. Box 5224
Sherman Oaks, CA 91413

Many childbirth-preparation groups offer much more than instruction in labor techniques. They have special classes for those needing only a "refresher course," book-lending services, parent hot lines, rap groups, teacher-training classes, separate cesarean-birth groups, newsletters, physician referral services, and infant-care classes. If you cannot afford the charges of any classes (customarily from $25 to $75), inquire about scholarships, which are frequently available.

Preparing for a cesarean birth

Parents whose infants will be born by cesarean surgery need different kinds of information and preparation. Standard preparation classes are inadequate because the breathing and relaxation techniques and long explanations of labor have little applicability to surgical procedures. Even the exercise programs may be inadequate for cesarean mothers; most important for them are those exercises that can help during recovery from the surgery.

Nevertheless, some cesarean mothers use Lamaze breathing techniques during surgery if they are awake but nervous.

Cesarean parents need to know about the actual operation, the role the father can play during birth, the usual length of the hospital stay, and time of recovery; and they need to explore their feelings about abdominal delivery, the difficulties of breast-feeding after surgery, the possibilities of family-centered maternity care, and much more.

Fortunately, cesarean support groups have sprung up all over the country. If you cannot find one in your community, or if you would simply like more information, write to C/SEC Inc., 66 Christopher Road, Waltham, MA 02154. This group not only distributes literature nationally but also has affiliated groups across the country.

A word about Leboyer births

To one physician, Dr. Frederick Leboyer, prepared childbirth was not the complete answer. He saw the unhappy faces of newborns and wondered if they were suffering after moving from the womb to the world outside. To some experts, who feel that newborns aren't sensitive to their surroundings, this concern seemed preposterous. But Leboyer reasoned that birth is at least as arduous a process for the infant as it is for the mother and that the sudden, final departure from the womb is traumatic enough without the horror of the blinding lights, unbearable sound, harsh fabric, icy temperatures, and metallic surfaces that greet our children as they enter the world.

Leboyer suggested easing the transition from womb to room by making the birth environment warm and less harshly lit, by eliminating noise, by leaving the umbilical cord intact until it stops pulsing, by placing the baby on the mother's abdomen directly after birth, by bathing the baby in warm, womb-temperature water, and by doing anything else possible to render the birthing atmosphere serene.

A Leboyer-style birth is not an alternative to prepared childbirth—it is a supplement. It can enhance the birth experience. There are, in addition, as many variations of this style of delivery as there are practitioners of it. Some physicians will even adapt it for a cesarean.

There are no classes offered in the Leboyer method. Parents and birth attendants who are interested in it can study Leboyer's slim book, *Birth Without Violence,* and adapt his ideas to their own situations and expectations.

If you need further information

In every community there is a surprisingly ample array of services available to expectant mothers and fathers:

• Local hospitals may have couples classes that instruct students in pregnancy, birth, and baby care; there are childbirth-preparation classes, tours of labor and delivery rooms, periodic lectures of interest to expectant parents. If you cannot afford outside preparation classes, a large hospital with a low-income clinic is sure to have free or reduced-rate classes. For parents seeking low-cost prenatal care, there are often hospital clinics for moderate-income families.

• Your nearest YMCA or JCC may be a valuable source of information about birth and baby-care resources, particularly if a toddler gym or swim class, which would tend to ensure the presence and interest of women who already have one or more children, is offered there. Check for special exercise and swim programs for expectant mothers, classes in baby care, and classes in any one of the aforementioned birth techniques.

• Community colleges may offer noncredit night courses in baby care, child psychology, parenthood, and birth preparation.

• Women's centers, besides offering low-cost or free pregnancy testing, may be able to refer you to physicians, recommend hospitals or childbirth instructors, and guide you to or help you organize a rap group for expectant mothers.

• Churches, yoga institutes, nutritionists, local La Leche League chapters, and even your community Red Cross may offer classes or groups aimed at expectant parents. Some organizations run twenty-four-hour hot lines for questions. County and municipal health departments may perform prenatal testing, administer vaccinations free of charge, or steer you to physicians, nurse-midwives, and childbirth instructors. Some may even lend you infant equipment.

• County medical societies can recommend physicians and often have a library or free phone messages on medical care, including medical aspects of pregnancy.

CHAPTER EIGHT
Having a Baby at Home

I don't know what I *expected* my home birth to be, but it *was* just fine. Afterwards, I felt, that's the way it should have been. I was satisfied, I was happy. I thought, everybody should do this! This is *right!*

—Mother recalling the home birth
of her second child

It wasn't momentous, it was lovely. During labor I wore my old bathrobe and slippers. I went downstairs to the kitchen and my mother made me and my husband hot chocolate. When the contractions got really hard, I lay down with my pillows and my down comforter. I wasn't afraid to shout and complain, because I knew no one would be rushing over with anesthetics. When I was ready to deliver, my husband was right there with me, and when Tessa was born, we held her for hours and hours, even my sons.

—Mother recalling the home birth
of her third child

Most American babies—99 percent by one reckoning—are born in hospitals, but there is a growing movement today toward home birth. According to Barb Barasa, a childbirth educator and proponent of home birth, in some counties of California 10 percent of all babies are born at home, by choice. The incidence of home birth, according to David Stewart of NAPSAC, has more than doubled in at least a dozen states in the last two to three years.

The interest stems from a disillusionment with hospitals and traditional obstetric care. Belatedly, hospitals are becoming more humane, but the grievances parents cite are still widespread and, many think, endemic to any kind of birth experience in a highly technological environment. Parents say that the sacrifices hospitals demand for the sake of efficiency and sterility are too great and sometimes actually harmful. They say that what is precisely most important about birth—safety, family togetherness, and familiar environment—can be realized better in a home setting. Finally, home-birth advocates believe that the whole orientation of the hospital toward sickness, disease, and medicine makes more likely the use of medical procedures that may not be needed. Some of the examples cited:

• *Routine unnecessary intervention.* There is no standard hospital procedure for the management of labor and birth. Hospital policies vary, as do physicians' instructions. Yet, some common procedures include:

1. *Anesthesia,* which can have deleterious effects on the baby.
2. *Shaving and enema.*
3. *Fetal monitoring,* an increasingly popular procedure for recording fetal heart rate and uterine contractions. While fetal monitoring is not used in all births by all hospitals, many practitioners are beginning to discuss its value in monitoring all births. Home-birth advocates, however, have pointed out that the fetal monitor may become a substitute for attentive, active human care. They say that use of the monitor can result in a higher cesarean birth rate because some birth attendants read the monitor incorrectly and mistakenly conclude that some babies are distressed.
4. *Forceps,* often used when an anesthetized mother cannot push effectively.
5. *Episiotomy.*
6. *IV's.*
7. *Cesarean birth,* undoubtedly a lifesaver when needed, although some observers are alarmed that the cesarean birth rate in some hospitals has climbed to 40 percent of all deliveries. In defense of the high rate, many physicians point out that surgery minimizes injury to the infant as well.
8. *Artificial rupture of membranes to speed labor.*

These procedures either will not be used or are less likely to be implemented during a home birth. Reporting to the March 1977 NAPSAC convention, Dr. Mayer Eisenstein, vice-president of the American College of Home Obstetrics, stated that in his home-birth practice during 1976, out of 300 births, the incidence of episiotomy was 2 percent, 4 percent of the mothers were transferred to the hospital, and the incidence of cesarean birth was 2 percent.

Of course, there is no guarantee that any woman can safely deliver at home. For her health and that of her baby, transfer to a hospital may be crucial. Once there, she may have to be shaved and have an IV and fetal monitor attached. She may have to undergo a cesarean section, forceps delivery, or episiotomy. But women who object to these procedures for normal, healthy births feel the chances of their being left to deliver without intervention are greatest at home.

• *Environment.* The stereotypical hospital birth starts with leaving a warm bed or house and dashing to the hospital (add hasty baby-sitting arrangements when needed). It proceeds with labor in a tiny cubicle and winds up in a bright, machine-filled delivery room. Some couples don't mind the change. They even rather enjoy the excitement. Others would just as soon stay at home and avoid the rush. Some researchers say that labor is much easier in a familiar environment. Finally, and perhaps most important, many women feel helpless or isolated in a hospital; rather than delivering, they "are delivered." At home, they feel central to the experience and very much cared for. Many have said they feel the birth experience is their own and not the hospital staff's.

• *Birth position.* Most women giving birth in hospitals deliver in the lithotomy (flat-on-the-back) position, with their feet up in stirrups. It is uncomfortable and more difficult to give birth in this position, although many physicians find it easier to see and manage births this way. In an often-quoted statement, Dr. Roberto Caldeyro-Barcia, president of the International Federation of Gynecologists and Obstetricians, said, "Except for being hanged by the feet, the supine position is the worst conceivable position for labor and delivery." At home, you usually deliver in bed, in any position you wish: squatting, sitting, on all fours, lying on your side.

• *Choice of participants.* While it is true most hospitals permit the baby's father in the labor and delivery rooms, he is usually the *only* one permitted to accompany the mother. Some couples wish to share the birth experience with other members of the family or friends, and it is rare for a hospital to permit this extra participation.

• *Other children.* Most mothers and children find it difficult to be apart for a three-to-seven-day hospital stay, although some hospitals do have sibling visitation programs. As a result of a long separation, children may be more alienated from a new sibling than they would have been if the mother had not left them for the birth. While some mothers actually permit older children to witness their home births, others say that just having older children in the same house, present right after the birth, made adjustment to the new infant easier for the whole family.

• *Separation from infant.* Many parents are uneasy or distraught about being separated from their newborns, a standard hospital procedure. Even if hospital policy permits ten minutes or even an hour or more of togetherness immediately after birth, some parents are opposed to the restriction and feel deprived of their child. In a home birth, of course, parents may hold the child as long as they wish.

• *Cost.* Your charges for a home birth include the physician's or midwife's fee, normal laboratory costs for pre- and postnatal tests, and the costs of equipment and supplies you must assemble. (Any of the home-birth groups listed on page 100 will be happy to inform you what supplies are necessary for a home birth.) The hospital bill for mother and newborn—the costliest part of hospital birth—is eliminated. Depending on the midwife's or physician's fee, a home birth may save you a third or even more.

Safety of home birth

By far the most frequently asked question about home birth is: "Is it safe?" Because most of us know little about birth and are so accustomed to linking the experience with hospitalization, the hospital seems the "natural" and safe place for mothers and infants. In addition, we hear stories of emergency situations that arise during childbirth, or know of women who had cesarean births, and we wonder how these would have been managed had the woman elected to have a home birth.

On one side of the home-birth question is the medical establishment: physicians, nurses, and hospitals. Many maintain that home birth can be unsafe, or, at any rate, that its safety has not yet been proved. The executive board of the American College of Obstetricians and Gynecologists issued this statement in May 1975 and reaffirmed it in May 1976:

Labor and delivery, while a physiologic process, clearly presents potential hazards to both mother and fetus before and after birth. These hazards require standards of safety which are provided in the hospital setting and cannot be matched in the home situation.

We recognize, however, the legitimacy of the concern of many that the events surrounding birth be an emotionally satisfying experience for the family. The College supports those actions that improve the experience of the family while continuing to provide the mother and her infant with accepted standards of safety available only in the hospital.

Dr. Richard Aubry, chairman of District II of the ACOG, amplified this position. He explained to a NAPSAC convention:

[The in-hospital setting] has allowed for optimal availability of blood transfusion, early diagnosis and treatment of infection, prompt response to unexpected maternal complications, as well as quickly available clinical, laboratory, radiology, anesthesia, and other consultative support services. More recently, the hospital setting has provided the additional fetal and neonatal safeguards of fetal monitoring and special neonatal resuscitation and intensive care.

Dr. Aubry also pointed to the improvement in maternal and fetal mortality statistics during the past few decades. He said that the improvement can be attributed to the high standards the ACOG has instituted for prenatal and hospital care.

Opposing this position are a number of home-birth advocates—parents, physicians, midwives, and nurses—who have joined forces to try to change the institution of birth in the United States. Such national groups as NAPSAC, Home Oriented Maternity Experience, and Association for Childbirth at Home, International (addresses at the end of this chapter), organize and disseminate information about alternative birth arrangements. They take issue with the supposition that the hospital is safer than the home for childbirth. They say that routine obstetric interventions all carry risks, and question the necessity of these risks for a woman in the midst of a normal labor or delivery. Some people also point out that in a hospital it is difficult for a woman to reject these procedures if she so wishes.

Home-birth advocates also point to such negative features of hospital births as the possibilities of staph infection in hospital nurseries, babies made groggy and unresponsive by medication administered to the mother, and rigid feeding schedules that cause infants and mothers distress—features that may not make hospitals the "safest" places to give birth.

It is important for all parents contemplating home birth, however, to consider the risks. True, most problems can be anticipated and avoided through good prenatal care and a careful screening program. Emergencies, however, arise—emergencies that cannot be handled at home. They include severe postpartum bleeding, cord prolapse, fetal distress, poor progress in labor, last-minute malpresentation, and meconium (mi-ko'-nee-um) staining (expulsion of fetal waste into the amniotic fluid, which may signal distress and which may be inhaled by the baby). In such cases, transfer to a hospital is imperative, and time and distance may be a factor.

Minimizing the risks

To reduce the risks of home birth, couples should have a skilled birth attendant, one who is:

- skilled in normal birth
- skilled at recognizing and handling problems
- skilled in home birth

If you have been able to find a physician or certified nurse-midwife who delivers at home, you may want to ask, in addition to the questions posed in Chapter 2:

1. *How many home deliveries have you attended? At how many were you assisting, and at how many were you the supervising attendant?*
2. *Under what circumstances would I be transferred to a hospital?*
3. *To what hospital would I be transferred should these complications arise?*
4. *Who would be my physician in the hospital? Would you accompany me? If not, who would be my advocate in the hospital?*

If you are considering having a lay midwife attend your birth, be aware of the limitations: lay midwives are not associated with hospitals and cannot legally dispense or prescribe medication. In many states, lay midwifery is outlawed or greatly restricted, so that your attendant may be operating illegally.

The other important way to minimize risk in home birth is careful screening. This is the responsibility of the birth attendant. Home-birth advocates have never maintained that *all* women can deliver out of the hospital; and *high-risk mothers cannot.* Estimates of the number of women who cannot (that is, those who will experience complications) run as high as 1 in 10.

To find that 1 in 10 (as nearly as possible), trained home-birth practitioners screen candidates very closely (any attendant who doesn't should not be retained). They will likely refuse to assist you at home if you have any of the following in your background: previous cesarean birth, hypertension, epilepsy, active venereal disease, heart or kidney disease, diabetes, severe anemia, Rh problems.

Sometimes home-birth attendants also have nonmedical criteria for accepting home-birth clients. Janet Epstein, a CNM with Maternity Center Associates in Washington, D.C., a practice that attends home births, says, in *Twenty-first Century Obstetrics Now!*, that these criteria include living a certain distance from a hospital, being willing to transfer to a hospital if the birth attendant so advises, agreeing to have a pediatrician examine the newborn, and attending childbirth-preparation classes.

Home birth: for you?

Who is giving birth at home? It seems the movement embraces a wide range of families—those birthing for the first time, those having second or later children, those who had poor hospital experiences, and those who had no major complaints in hospitals. Some couples view birth as calm and routine; others invite many friends and relatives to the "event." The only thing that these families have in common is a commitment to humane childbirth. And it is fair to say, too, that most home-birth families, far from being back-to-nature zealots, are conventional families who have studied risks and benefits, thought carefully about their future child, and made the decision that seemed best for them.

For the vast majority of American women, of course, home birth is not the best decision. They are comfortable and secure in a hospital environment; they feel assured knowing there is emergency treatment easily available should the need arise. To them, the hospital is the natural place to give birth, and they regard the sacrifices as inconvenient but necessary.

Is there an answer? Need there be? The wide range of options beginning to be available to expectant parents in this country is exciting. Those affiliated with obstetrics—from physicians to midwives—should realize the roots of this diversity: the search by parents and professionals for a safe and meaningful mode of childbirth. If our childbirth professionals can aid parents by working together to achieve these goals, the controversies that now rage may fade away.

If you need more information on home birth, write to:

David Stewart
National Association of
Parents and Professionals
for Safe Alternatives
in Childbirth (NAPSAC)
P.O. Box 267
Marble Hill, MO 63764

Home Oriented Maternity
Experience (HOME)
511 New York Avenue
Takoma Park,
Washington, D.C. 20012

Association for Childbirth
at Home, International (ACHI)
Box 1219
Cerritos, CA 90701

Home Opportunity for the
Pregnancy Experience
(HOPE)
P.O. Box 78
Wauconda, IL 60084

CHAPTER NINE
When You're over Thirty

Anyone sitting in an obstetrician's waiting room quickly notices them: the surprising number of pregnant women in their thirties and even forties. If a fast survey were taken, it would no doubt reveal that many of these patients—some old enough to be parents of teenagers—were pregnant for the first time.

Every demographic study confirms the fact that women are waiting longer to start their families. Even those who marry at twenty may wait ten years to have a baby. The need to build a career, the high rate of divorce and remarriage, and even peer pressure may postpone pregnancy a decade or longer. Ambitious and realistic couples have become aware of the limitations and problems posed by the baby they have too early.

Rational reasons for delaying pregnancy submerge the issue, but eventually it resurfaces—often when a woman nears or reaches thirty. Articles about the health problems of older women and their babies force many of us to adopt a "now-or-never" philosophy around that age. The sentiments of Theresa, a twenty-nine-year-old stockbroker, are repeated in countless conversations: "If I'm ever going to have a baby, it had better be soon. I'm just getting too old."

Are these fears and self-inflicted pressures sensible? What's it like having a baby after age thirty? Are the problems just too overwhelming and the medical risks too grave? Or is it true, as many women in their late thirties are now saying, that later motherhood is terrific?

Medical considerations

Most women thirty and older who contemplate pregnancy are concerned with possible medical problems that may occur because of their age. They worry that they'll have trouble conceiving, that their baby will have a chromosomal disorder such as Down's syndrome, that labor and delivery will be much harder for them than for a younger woman. These concerns are understandable; traditionally, medical experts have emphasized the risks involved in delaying a pregnancy (especially the first) until after the mother turns thirty. But many physicians now feel that "older" mothers have had an undeserved reputation for increased difficulties during pregnancy, labor, and delivery. Today, as regards pregnancy, maternal age alone is not considered so important as a woman's health history and the quality of medical care she receives. Let's look at some medical aspects of having a baby past thirty.

• *Fertility.* Any woman who wants to have a baby may have trouble conceiving. But fertility problems—which may take a considerable amount of time to correct—are of special concern to women over thirty because they have fewer years remaining for childbearing. Though many women continue to ovulate until they are fifty or older, the supply of viable eggs does diminish with age. Whether this general decline in fertility begins at thirty or thirty-five is subject to debate. Most studies, however, agree that after a woman turns forty the decline is pronounced. (It should be noted that male fertility declines more gradually than female fertility, and some men in their seventies and even eighties are capable of fathering children.)

In addition to the reduction of eggs that comes with age, a woman's fertility may be impaired simply because her body has had a longer time to be exposed to infections that can damage her ovaries, uterus, or Fallopian tubes. If these organs are structurally imperfect, correction may be long overdue and thus more difficult. Male infertility may occur when sperm are not produced in sufficient quantity, or are not mature enough to achieve fertilization, or are unable to meet the egg. Again, infection, structural problems, and even drug intake are some of the factors that affect sperm production. The older the man, the more likely the damage, if any. Inability to conceive can also result from a combination of minor problems in both partners.

Since time is of the essence for a woman over thirty, how long should she wait before seeking help with a possible fertility problem? Some specialists suggest that couples try to conceive for six months before looking into professional help. But if the woman usually has had irregular menstrual cycles, or if either partner was previously married and tried to conceive without success, the pair should probably start checking into their fertility right away and receive complete physical examinations.

•*Genetics.* Having a child with Down's syndrome is probably the major worry of women over thirty who want to become pregnant. A fetus affected by Down's syndrome (or mongolism) has an extra chromosome, which results in mental and physical retardation. The incidence of Down's syndrome in the fetus increases with maternal age, regardless of whether it is a woman's first or fifth pregnancy. (A few other chromosomal disorders are linked to maternal age, but they occur less frequently than Down's syndrome, which strikes about six thousand newborns each year.) Only 1 woman in about 2,000 at age twenty will bear a child with Down's syndrome. At thirty, the statistics rise to 1 in about 1,000; at thirty-five, 1 in about 400; at forty, 1 in about 100; at forty-five, 1 in about 40.

How does the mother's age relate to the incidence of Down's syndrome? A woman's immature eggs are present in her body even before her birth. As she gets older, so do the eggs—and at some point their quality will diminish. Years of contact with radiation, drugs, and other chemicals may also increase the chances that the eggs of older women will be damaged.

What about paternal age? Does it have any effect on the quality of sperm? Though men do become less fertile with age, sperm are produced continuously throughout a man's reproductive years. For this reason, many experts feel that it's less likely the sperm will contribute the extra chromosome that characterizes Down's syndrome. Some specialists, however, do recommend genetic counseling and possibly amniocentesis if the father is fifty-five or older. Regardless of his age, if a man knows of chromosomal disorders in his family, has previously fathered a child (even by another woman) with a chromosomal problem, or has a previous wife who suffered several miscarriages, he should seek out genetic counseling before another pregnancy is initiated.

•*Amniocentesis.* Today, pregnant women who are concerned about Down's syndrome because of their age or genetic background can undergo amniocentesis to determine the health of the fetus. Amniocentesis is generally a simple and safe procedure: a sample of amniotic fluid is withdrawn from the uterus at fourteen to sixteen weeks of pregnancy, then analyzed in a laboratory. (For a complete discussion of this procedure, see page 52.) This analysis can disclose Down's syndrome, as well as many other chromosomal and hereditary diseases in the fetus. Amniocentesis can bring some peace of mind to women who undergo the procedure. Ninety-five percent of those who have the test learn that Down's syndrome or other abnormalities are not present in the fetus. Couples who learn that the fetus *is* affected can begin to make preparations for having the child, or they may opt for a second-trimester abortion.

Although the incidence of Down's syndrome begins to rise slightly after a woman reaches thirty, most doctors do not recommend routine amniocentesis for patients under thirty-five. At thirty-five, the risk of having an affected child increases sharply. (Of course, a couple's genetic background may suggest other reasons for having the test even before the pregnant woman is thirty-five.) According to some medical experts, not all women who *should* be informed *are* informed by their physicians about amniocentesis. But doctors may soon have a legal responsibility to offer patients the option of amniocentesis, depending on the outcome of cases now in court.

• *Miscarriage.* The chances of miscarrying seem to increase as a woman gets older, especially after she reaches thirty-five, perhaps because older women are more likely to carry defective embryos (that is, with chromosomal abnormalities). Maternal problems, such as damage to reproductive organs from previous births, abortions, and surgery, may also precipitate miscarriage, and are more likely to occur in older women. Nevertheless, the health of the mother's reproductive system, not the age of the mother, is the overriding consideration in whether a pregnancy will continue to term.

• *Multiple births.* Older women who want to become, or are, pregnant frequently hear that they're more likely to have twins because of their age. Age, along with race, heredity, and the number of previous children, does influence the chances that a couple will naturally produce nonidentical twins, triplets, and quadruplets. (The frequency of identical twins, triplets, and so on, does not seem to be influenced by these factors.)

The chance of having a multiple pregnancy is greatest when a woman is thirty-five to forty. After age forty, the incidence of twinning is lower. Experts say, however, that the influence of parity (number of other children) on twinning cannot be totally separated from the influence of age. Women of thirty-five who are pregnant for the first time, rather than the fourth, run a smaller chance of producing twins.

Also, women with fertility problems may be using drugs to conceive, which will increase their chances of having a multiple pregnancy. More than one fetus is a strain on any woman's system. Multiple pregnancies mean the mother and fetus must be more closely watched for possible complications. But, all things being equal, older pregnant women should not suffer more discomforts from multiple pregnancy merely because of their age.

• *Course of pregnancy, labor, and delivery.* In the past, many doctors discouraged older women from becoming pregnant, theorizing the risks and discomforts were too great. Today, that kind of advice is rare. Older pregnant women follow the same regimen as others (except for amniocentesis). Increasingly, medical experts are seeing that there is no ideal age to be pregnant, and a woman who is healthy can most likely have a successful pregnancy and delivery regardless of how old she is. Problems that may develop during pregnancy, such as toxemia, hypertension, and kidney disease, are seen as not specifically related to maternal age, but dependent more on the mother's general health, nutrition, and medical history.

Statistically, older women delivering a first child tend to have slightly longer labors than younger women do. (Age does not seem to affect the length of subsequent labors and deliveries unless there have been many years between births.) Throughout the years, most studies have reported that the incidence of cesarean birth increases with the age of the mother (physicians we spoke to, however, noted no difference in the cesarean rate of their older and younger patients). This apparent increase may occur because labors tend to be longer, or placenta previa more common in older mothers—two situations that may indicate a need for a cesarean. More frequent cesareans may also result because many physicians automatically regard the over-thirty pregnancy as high-risk, one in which vaginal delivery is more dangerous for the mother and the baby.

Your attitude is different, too

We've discussed elsewhere how pregnancy is a psychological as well as a physical state, and this is true for women of any age.

Yet certain feelings and sensibilities are unique to the older pregnant woman. Lodged at a position in life significantly different from that reached by a twenty-year-old, for example, the older mother-to-be associates pregnancy with a special range of problems and possibilities.

Just *becoming* pregnant, for example—something a younger woman may take for granted—can be a monumental experience. Years of trying to conceive, or the simple knowledge that fertility declines with age, can make conception a feat in itself, an almost magical occurrence. Even if a couple has been using birth control for years, it is reassuring and surprisingly pleasant for a woman to discover that her body is working the way it should.

Older women may be less ambivalent about wanting a baby, and more positive about the whole experience of pregnancy. After having logged so much time at a job or done extensive traveling, they may be very comfortable with the idea of being "tied down." The outside world seems less glamorous, easily escapable. One thirty-six-year-old mother of twin toddlers, a former stewardess, said, "Maybe I just got cynical. But by the time I was thirty, I no longer found my job exciting or felt the need to define myself by it. When the twins were born, I left flying without looking back."

A woman who has been a success in her career is less apt to wonder "what might have been" had she not become pregnant. Besides, financial security, years spent cultivating the relationship with her partner, comfortable and secure living arrangements, and sturdy friendships all go a long way toward reducing the stresses of pregnancy for an older mother. Those expecting a second or subsequent child benefit incalculably from having been down the road before.

Older expectant mothers and fathers usually enjoy another aspect of pregnancy: an improved relationship with their siblings and parents. Brothers and sisters with kids of their own may consider that the parents-to-be have now "arrived," and share their concerns with them more readily. The new parents may have more to share as well, and may be eager to introduce their baby to his/her cousins. At the same time, couples whose parents had long ago given up on grandchildren may be cheered by the commotion a newborn is bound to create.

Working through problems

Despite the many advantages of older motherhood, there is a negative side. An older mother may be more likely to worry about her baby's health, even if her fears are groundless. She may be aware that the incidence of Down's syndrome and other chromosomal disorders increases with the age of the mother. Possibly, she's heard stories about the difficult labor and delivery experiences some older women have had. It helps to know exactly how great the odds are for a good pregnancy, normal delivery, and healthy baby. Amniocentesis, when indicated, can go a long way toward calming apprehensions.

The uniqueness of her situation—for example, finding herself the only thirty-seven-year-old in the maternity shop—can be amusing, delightful, or frustrating. A woman may look younger than she really is while she's pregnant. But at times, the older mother may feel isolated. Some of her friends may be focusing on the problems of adolescents, while she is concerned about breastfeeding. Yet she may also feel out of touch with the much younger pregnant women she encounters at prepared-childbirth classes.

Pregnancy is an important time to share experiences and feelings with other women; it pays to make the effort to find other expectant parents with whom you can feel open and comfortable. Alternatively, share your thoughts with friends who have children. All women remember their pregnancies, no matter how many years have passed. Old friends can be a vital source of support.

Your life will change—and you know it

Every family undergoes change with the addition of a baby—and parental age merely affects the kinds, not the quantity, of adjustments. Older couples, entrenched for years in a comfortable, easygoing routine, may be apprehensive about giving that up. They worry about having the stamina to keep up with an energetic toddler. They may look wistfully at their furnishings, antiques, plants, and pets, and silently catalog the losses. Even converting a study to a nursery can be somewhat upsetting for a woman who has long treasured a quiet, isolated workroom.

Couples long accustomed to two hefty incomes may also need to adjust their material expectations. If one parent will be giving up work outside the home, they may have to curtail cleaning help, frequent dinners out, expensive vacations, or other "luxuries" that have come to seem more like necessities. Even if both parents continue to hold outside jobs, a good housekeeper means a big chunk of someone's take-home pay.

If these worries absorb you, relax. Everyone, not just the older parent, must come to grips with the changes a baby means. Good planning, the free flow of ideas between expectant parents, and a honest, ongoing reexamination of your priorities really helps. You are never locked into a life-style. As one forty-two-year-old father said, "When Judy was pregnant, I was extremely concerned about maintaining our old life—traveling, the best clothes, restaurants—after the baby came. Since Jeremy's birth, though, I've found that my priorities have changed. I'm less concerned about material things and more concerned about intangibles like love and the time I need to be a good parent."

You and your partner

If you've been married for many years, you may find the stability and long familiarity a blessing during the nine months of pregnancy, and afterward. On the other hand, if your husband is at or approaching the peak of his career, he may have little time to give you the support you need. You may justifiably find yourself wondering whether your having a baby will cap a long, rewarding relationship or cause it to crumble.

Outside jobs—yours and your partner's—can also be a significant source of conflict during pregnancy. If you and your mate have both reached responsible positions, you may at times feel resentful if your partner continues to advance, while you make plans to stay home and care for the baby. If both your jobs require much after-five attention, you may wonder about ways to meet those needs, as well as the demands of a young child.

Fathers need to examine their feelings, too. While having a child can often be an asset in the world of work (you may seem more the "solid citizen"), it's important to consider your emotional needs as well. Some older fathers-to-be worry about "losing" their wives, especially if there have just been the two of them for many years. Others do swift calculations ("When I'm fifty, my child will only be six") and worry about how their future son or daughter will like having a much older father.

These are all normal concerns, and rarely insurmountable. Expectant parents need time to consider new approaches to job, marriage, friends, and family. If you are committed to having a baby, you will find ways to adjust your needs and priorities to the reality.

The practical side

On the job

• Chances are you've been immersed in your career for at least a decade, with a twelve-hour day and working weekends a fact of

life. Now that you are pregnant, however, realize that you'll probably need more rest than you're accustomed to getting. It will be
hard to cut down at first, but the strains that pregnancy places on
your body, combined with the pace of a high-pressure job, may
exhaust you. Early in pregnancy, begin to normalize your hours
and try to decrease your co-workers' expectations of you.

• Along with cutting back to a livable schedule, realize that you
owe it to yourself to enjoy this pregnancy and to prepare for your
baby. If you've waited a long time to be pregnant, consider taking
time off to appreciate the experience. Plunge into the expectant-
parent routine. Although you may initially be perplexed or slightly
impatient with childbirth-preparation classes, medical appointments, and tours of the hospital, get involved! Plan your schedule
to include these activities, and more. You'll find the time well
spent and the childbirth experience enhanced for your efforts. And
you'll also be alleviating feelings of isolation.

• You don't have to set an example for your employees. Nor
should you push yourself to assert your ability. Work at a comfortable pace and let your productivity speak for itself. Incidentally, if you are puzzled about when and how to tell employees of
your pregnancy, just remember that the decision is yours alone.
Exercise the same discretion that you would for any other personal
matter.

• Take a long look at your job's fringe benefits. Lots of accrued
vacation time? See if you can use it for an extended postpartum
leave. Worried about losing seniority? Generally you can't, but
check with the personnel office. If you've really established a foot-
hold at your office, you may be able to arrange flexible hours or
part-time employment after the baby's birth. One magazine writer
did all her work at home for three months after her daughter's
birth, then returned to her job three days a week until the baby
was two.

• Look out for your own best interests. If you are tempted to ask
your secretary to perform more of your work or run a lot of personal errands simply because you are too tired, ask yourself if your
job is becoming burdensome. Perhaps you should consider cutting
back. If your work involves frequent traveling, plan to ease up in
the later months. If entertaining responsibilities invariably involve
alcohol and cigarettes, don't hesitate to change the focus to avoid
these toxic substances.

At home

• In the first flush of motherhood, you may be tempted to charge out to a house in the suburbs. Don't. You've logged long years in the city and you're comfortable there. You might be disappointed if you indulge your fantasies. And at least for the first year, when a child doesn't need a green lawn or friends down the block, stick to familiar surroundings where you'll have the comfort of established routines, familiar faces and services, and stimulating surroundings.

• Thinking about moving closer to family? Take time to make that decision. If you've long lived independently, it may mean an enormous readjustment to return to the fold. Adapting to motherhood is difficult enough without the added burden of figuring out your role as a daughter or sister at the same time.

• Unless you *must* move, stay where you have good friends, at least for the first few months postpartum. The value of this kind of stability is immeasurable, especially for couples used to relying on supportive friends.

You are not too old

The physicians we spoke with when we prepared this chapter agreed that age alone should not be a factor in deciding on a pregnancy. "If an older woman *can* conceive, and there are no medical problems, I would never discourage her from having a baby," said one. That's good news for all of us because it means many more options are available when deciding on the best way to arrange personal lives and careers. With health—not age—the deciding factor for pregnancy, and with prenatal tests available to help us determine the well-being of the fetus, women need no longer feel locked into jobs, marriages, or relationships that lead to "babies by age thirty." Instead, we're all freer to consider the possibilities of parenthood carefully and to take full advantage of other paths open to us.

CHAPTER TEN
What You Will Need for Your Baby

If you've never outfitted a baby or nursery before, the number and variety of baby furnishings are bewildering. New parents rarely know exactly what they will need and which items are less than useful. If the range of options seems confusing, the information that follows will help you to understand infant paraphernalia better.

All new parents should have a copy of the *Consumer's Union Guide to Buying for Babies* (Warner Books). It's got a wealth of information on baby equipment, including data on safety, convenience, and value. In addition, the Consumer Product Safety Commission, listed in the telephone directory under United States Government, has literature on baby product safety, and the Juvenile Products Manufacturers Association, 66 East Main Street, Moorestown, NJ 08057, has leaflets and other materials on baby furnishings.

Sometime after the first trimester, expectant parents should begin thinking about what they will need for the baby immediately after birth. Although some parents delay stocking a nursery until after delivery, you'd be wise to prepare as much as you can before the baby comes—it's unlikely you'll have much time afterward. Even the most organized parents run themselves ragged at first, dashing out for diapers, or a thermometer, or extra stretch suits. You certainly won't have time to do major buying, to check garage sales, or to comparison-shop.

The lists in this chapter enumerate only the things you should assemble before birth. Eventually, you'll be shopping for more paraphernalia: playpen, high chair, booster seat, and toys. But these are the basics you should acquire now.

Furnishings

The basics for a newborn are:

- crib and mattress
- changing table
- infant seat
- bathing equipment
- bumper guards
- infant car carrier
- basket or bag for soiled laundry
- dresser or bins for clothes storage
- plastic pail for cloth diapers, or plastic-bag-lined wastebasket for disposables
- carryall for outings

• *Crib and mattress.* A tiny infant doesn't need a crib at first; it can, of course, sleep in a padded dresser drawer, carriage, basket, or bassinet. But the baby *will* need a crib by about the age of six weeks so you might just as well get one before birth, set it up, and slowly accustom your baby to what will be its surroundings for about the next two and a half years. Families with pets and toddlers, particularly, prefer cribs to less protective enclosures.

All new cribs are constructed according to 1973 federal safety standards. Cribs have single- or double-drop sides (a question of convenience), and extras such as spindles, decals, and designs.

If you are purchasing a used crib, however, find one that meets current standards. This may take some searching. The Consumer Product Safety Commission estimates that there are eleven million cribs in use that do not meet these standards:

• Crib slats must be no more than two and three-eighths inches apart (about the width of three adult fingers) to keep an infant from wriggling its body through the slats until its head gets caught.

• A mattress must fit snugly into the crib. If you have room for two fingers between mattress and crib, the mattress is too small. A baby can suffocate if it wedges itself between mattress and crib. (If your mattress is in good condition but small, you can stuff rolled towels into the space between it and the crib frame.)

• Hook the mattress support on its lowest position. With the crib side *up,* the distance between the mattress support and the top of the drop side should be twenty-six inches. Hook the mattress support on its highest position. With the crib side lowered, the top of the drop side should be at least nine inches above the mattress support.

• All wooden surfaces should be smooth and splinter-free; paint should be nontoxic; teething rails should be secure.
• All hardware should be free of sharp or rough edges.
• Latches on drop sides should be secure to prevent accidental release. They should require two actions (for example, pulling up the side, then kicking the foot release) to drop.

• *Changing table.* You can buy a changing table or make one. Any high surface—dresser, sink side, or table—with a cushioned, waterproof pad on top will do. If the surface is too low, you'll find yourself bending too much, straining your back muscles. Be sure that the changing table has adequate room to store or hold everything you'll need for changing: diapers, cloth wipes, ointments, pins, new clothes. Everything must be at hand so that you don't have to leave the infant unattended. The advantages of purchasing a new changing table are that you can obtain one equipped with safety belt and guardrails or one with a recessed rather than a flat top. (But no matter which type you use, *never leave a baby unattended on a changing table.*) Families who live in two-story residences may need a changing table on both floors.

• *Infant seat.* If you enjoy your baby's company (and vice versa), an infant seat is a necessity. You prop up the baby in the seat, strap it in, and set the seat on any low, wide, nonskid surface (couch, floor, coffee table) so that s/he can watch what's going on. Not all carriers, however, are safe. Each year, hospital emergency rooms see about a thousand accidents caused by these seats. Be sure, when purchasing one, that:
• It has a wide, sturdy base to avoid tipping.
• It has a safety belt or a place to attach a harness.
• It has a nonslip bottom.
• The support device cannot collapse.
• It is constructed from sturdy material, not flimsy, breakable plastic.

• *Bathing equipment.* You can sponge-bathe newborns for a while, but eventually you'll want to introduce your infant to a tub bath. Any wide plastic or enameled basin will do. It's especially handy if you can set the tub near a sink. In fact, some mothers use the sink itself for bathing their infants.

• **Bumper guards.** These fit around the crib's perimeter and keep infants from bumping against slats. Be sure guards run around the entire crib and attach securely to the slats in at least six places. To prevent baby from chewing or swallowing ties, fasten them *outside* the crib and snip off excess material. If guards cannot be secured on the bottom, the infant can still push between the guard and the mattress. Bumper guards should surely be used in older cribs that do not have a two-and-three-eighths-inch spacing between slats.

• **Infant car carrier.** An infant car carrier is a reclining seat engineered to protect babies in the car. It is the only way to transport an infant safely. Regular infant seats (for feeding and carrying) are not designed for crash protection, and a baby can be wrenched from a parent's arms by the force of a collision.

Unfortunately, many of the carriers in use today are not as safe as they could be (and some are totally ineffective). A parent group, Action for Child Transportation Safety, has been fighting for tough safety standards. In May 1980, regulations from the Department of Transportation took effect. Parents should make sure that any seat they buy has been crash-tested successfully.

Many families purchase or inherit a used infant car carrier. This situation poses problems. If you haven't inherited the instructions as well, you may use the carrier incorrectly, completely canceling any safety benefits. You won't know if a previously owned seat is being used correctly unless you have that seat's instruction booklet. Write to the manufacturer to obtain it.

Having an instruction booklet is not enough. When purchasing or borrowing an *infant* carrier, remember that it must be designed to face the rear of the car, never the front. There should be a harness to secure the infant, and the carrier should be designed to strap to the seat with a lap belt. If the carrier is convertible (can be converted from infant to toddler use), be certain you have the parts and capability to top-anchor the seat if that should be necessary for the particular model (if the carrier requires a top anchor and you don't use it, you render the seat unsafe).

If you have questions about a seat you own or want to buy, write to: Physicians for Automotive Safety, P.O. Box 208, Rye, NY 10580. For fifty cents and a large stamped, self-addressed envelope, this organization will send the pamphlet *Don't Risk Your Child's Life!* about infant and toddler car seats.

Not necessary, but nice to have

• *Basket, bassinet, or cradle.* For newborns only. Not a necessity, but definitely an advantage if you live in a two-story house or if you'd like to keep the newborn by your bed at night. Some people believe that newborns prefer these smaller confines to the large, open spaces of a crib.

• *Front carrier.* Something like a rucksack, only worn in front and designed to hold babies. Some newborns enjoy long periods of quiet bliss when stuffed into a soft carrier; others can't stand the confinement. If you purchase a carrier, be sure of the following:
  • You know how to strap yourself in properly and how to seat your baby in the carrier.
  • It is comfortable for you and the infant, and convenient to put on and remove.
  • It matches your baby's size and weight.
  • Leg openings are small enough to prevent the baby from slipping out, yet big enough so that her/his thighs are not chafed.
  • The material is sturdy, and stitching is strong and intact. Check for frayed or torn areas, and be sure all straps, snaps, and seams are secure.

• *Portable crib, crib pen, specialty crib, travel crib.* These are non-full-size, sometimes collapsible cribs that are useful as second cribs or for travel (many motels and hotels, however, provide these free of charge). Any non-full-size crib (except mesh, net, and screen cribs, car beds, cradles, and bassinets) sold after August 10, 1976, must comply with safety standards similar to those applicable to full-size cribs:
  • The distance between the crib slats should be two and three-eighths inches.
  • The mattress should fit snugly.
  • When the mattress support is at the lowest position and the crib side is at its highest position, the side should measure at least twenty-two inches. When the mattress support is at its highest position and the crib side is at its lowest, the side should measure at least five inches.
  • Hardware and wooden surfaces should be smooth; latches on drop sides should be secure.

• *Carriage.* Expensive, bulky, and hard to store, a carriage is nevertheless a lovely thing to have for walking a baby. Sometimes a carriage can be useful, too, for walking a colicky infant around the house. It can double as a bassinet, and some carriages even convert to strollers. Check for the following when purchasing a carriage:

• Does the carriage tip over easily, or will it be stable no matter how actively the baby moves around inside? Large, sturdy wheels contribute to stability.

• Do the brakes hold securely? Four-wheel brakes are better than two-wheel brakes, and both are superior to one-wheel brakes.

• Does the carriage have effective guards against accidental collapse?

• Are all inside metal parts covered or cushioned?

• Is a safety harness included? If not, can a harness you purchase separately be attached?

• *Umbrella stroller.* These are the strollers you see everywhere: the ones that fold up easily, to be carried like an umbrella. Because they generally are light (about six pounds) and portable, they're perfect for shopping and traveling (you can even take them on a plane). Some people think they aren't comfortable for kids, but few children object to them for short trips. When purchasing, check the device that locks the stroller open. It should offer security against accidental collapse. Try to get a stroller that doesn't easily tip backward, and one with substantial, good-sized wheels. Again, two-wheel brakes are better than one-wheel brakes. A new generation of umbrella strollers is now available with hard-backed, reclining seats. These strollers are more expensive and heavier, but they may be more comfortable for your child.

Repairing used equipment

If you've inherited baby furnishings or equipment and are thinking about refurbishing, there are several steps you should take for safety. The Consumer Product Safety Commission and others recommend that you:

• Sand or scrape off old paint and refinish with lead-free, high-quality household enamel paint. Don't use paint manufactured before 1972, when many paints contained a higher percentage of lead than is permitted now.

• Purchase a harness and attach if there is no adequate restraining strap system.

• Repair latching and braking mechanisms.

• Cover sharp edges, latches, and bolts with heavy-duty vinyl tape.
• Remove cracked or splintered plastic pieces.

Infant clothing

• *Cold weather.* If your baby will be born during cold weather, you should have ready, before birth:

8–12 stretchies (terry-cloth-like suits with feet and long sleeves, equipped with snaps or zippers)
8 snap undershirts (twelve-month size)
4 blanket sleeper bags
1 knit sweater and leggings outfit
2–3 cardigan sweaters
1–2 knit hats
1 bunting, pram bag, or snowsuit (buntings and pram bags are snowsuits without legs)
4 pairs elasticized, heavy-knit booties

To dress a baby for an *outing,* you would layer as follows:

diaper and undershirt
stretchy
sweater and leggings
hat
bunting or snowsuit
heavy blanket

To dress a baby for *sleeping,* you would layer as follows:

diaper and undershirt
stretchy
blanket sleeper or receiving blanket plus heavy blanket

To dress a baby *during the day,* you would layer as follows:

diaper and undershirt
stretchy
sweater or receiving blanket if necessary

It's highly impractical and often a waste of time to "dress up" an infant, but if you've received gifts of clothes that you want to use (and we all do) and the outfits don't have feet, booties may be necessary to keep tiny feet warm.

• **Warm weather.** If your baby will be born in warm weather, you should have ready, before birth:

12 snap undershirts
8 short-sleeved light cotton gowns
1 lightweight sweater or jacket
4 terry, cotton or seersucker sleeveless jumpsuits
2 lightweight stretchies
sun hat
light cotton booties or socks

For daytime:

diaper and jumpsuit

For outdoors:

diaper and jumpsuit
hat
terry coverup to prevent sunburn
lightweight booties

For sleeping:

diaper and undershirt *or*
diaper and gown

Bedding

Acquire the following before your baby's birth:

4–6 soft cotton sheets
2 quilted mattress covers
4 large flannel-covered rubber pads
4 medium flannel-covered rubber pads
6 receiving blankets
3 heavy blankets or comforters, machine-washable
2 baby bath towels
6 baby washcloths

To make up the crib, you would layer over the mattress as follows:

    quilted mattress cover
    sheet
    rubber pad
    baby
    receiving blanket
    comforter or blanket

Receiving blankets are also excellent for wrapping the baby during the day, covering the changing-table top, holding under the baby during a bath, laying atop a car seat or stroller on a hot day.

Pharmaceuticals

Assemble these before your baby's birth:

    mild bar soap for baths
    petroleum jelly
    baby shampoo
    rubbing alcohol
    diaper rash ointment
    baby hairbrush
    2 pacifiers
    cotton balls
    2 packages moist wipes for outings
    blunt-edged nail scissors

If you plan to use cloth diapers, have on hand:

    3–4 dozen prefolded cloth diapers (or make arrangements with
        a diaper service)
    4 sets double-lock safety pins
    6 waterproof pants
    1 box newborn-size disposable diapers

If you plan to use disposables, have on hand:

    4–6 boxes newborn-size disposable diapers
    1 dozen cloth diapers (for burping, crib, and so on)

Feeding equipment

If you plan to breast-feed, have on hand:

2–4 plastic 8-ounce bottles plus caps and screw rings (bottles are needed for water, juice, or for occasional formula or expressed-milk feedings)
bottle-and-nipple brush
6–8 nipples
or
1 kit presterilized, disposable nursers (includes holders, disposable bottles, nipples, collars, caps)
2 extra nipples
nipple brush
nursing pads

If you plan to bottle-feed:

8–12 plastic 8-ounce bottles with caps and screw rings
12–16 nipples
sterilizer (electric or standard) or deep kettle
tongs
can opener
large measuring cup
bottle-and-nipple brush
or
1 kit presterilized disposable nursers
4 extra nipples
nipple brush

Do not stock formula until you know what brand your pediatrician customarily recommends.

CHAPTER ELEVEN
New Routines

Pregnancy does not alter the daily activities of some women; from conception to labor they carry on as always—working, gardening, traveling, sleeping, commuting. The extra weight doesn't tire them; physical discomforts are minimal. Many of these women, in fact, are surprised that anyone *would* make allowances or seek special considerations during this time.

For others, the discomforts of the first and third trimesters are bothersome. Traveling by air, jogging, taking care of other children—these activities may make you tired or uncomfortable, even if you've always been energetic. You may be surprised, and somewhat impatient, with your limited capacities; even sleeping can be difficult if you can't find a good position.

Besides the ways discomforts may alter your activities, pregnancy presents other considerations. We often ask ourselves during pregnancy: "Is what I'm doing safe for my baby?" You may wonder about the baby's safety while you're running or doing yoga. You may think about it while trying to sleep on your stomach or when traveling by plane. And you *should* consider it when you work with all the potent chemicals that fill household shelves: oven, drain, and all-purpose cleaners; pesticides; furniture refinishers; paints; aerosols; and more.

It's not difficult to be especially careful and aware of the things you do, touch, and ingest during pregnancy. It definitely is a time to refrain from performing certain activities and from using some products. But *which* ones? As a guide, try dividing the things you do and substances you come in contact with into two categories: things known to be harmful to the fetus, and things whose effects on the fetus are not known. By far, most of the substances we touch and ingest, and many of our activities, fall into the second category. But if you have doubts about any activity, food, or product, take the time to educate yourself and get the advice of your physician or midwife.

Commuting to your job

Many women would be happy to work outside the home right through the ninth month if it weren't for commuting. During rush hours, jammed buses and trains mean a lot of jostling, standing, and stuffiness. Getting to work may be more tiring than time spent on the job. So you may be forced to quit work, or take a leave of absence and lose the income, even if your job itself is not tiring or unpleasant.

To ease commuting problems, ask your employer if you may rearrange your schedule—to come in and leave an hour earlier, for example, so that you can avoid rush hours. If need be, negotiate a partial pay cut for reduced hours, take fifteen minutes off your lunch hour, or take work home; then use the extra time to commute during off-hours. (Don't skip lunch or breaks as a compromise. You need the food and the rest.) When presented with a forthright and unapologetic request, many employers will respond flexibly.

If you can't change your hours, but find commuting particularly tiring and uncomfortable (especially when you're nauseated), try to improve the circumstances. Don't run up flights of stairs or across several blocks to make a train or bus. If you're not used to sprinting, the exertion will tire you easily and you may need a while to recover. If you're particularly uncomfortable or feel faint, don't stand there and suffer, ask someone for a seat. You'll probably get one if you indicate you are ill. (Don't expect a seat to be *offered*. Many women say they were *never* offered a seat while commuting during pregnancy.)

Carry mints, which can help when you feel light-headed. Consider walking instead of standing in a slow-moving bus; physicians are unanimous on the benefits of walking. If you're feeling nauseated on a bus or train, try relaxed deep breathing, or bring crackers to chew. You might also carry a plastic sipper filled with ginger ale. The main consideration with nausea is not to travel on an empty stomach, a particular concern for the evening commute when your last meal may have been five hours earlier. A healthful snack at 3:00 P.M.—such as cheese with crackers—helps.

You can also use your commuting time for exercise. Try the Kegel exercises; rotating, flexing, and extending feet; deep breathing; graduated body relaxations; pelvic rock. (For descriptions of the Kegel exercises and pelvic rock, see page 158.)

Traveling during pregnancy

Many people believe that women shouldn't travel long distances during pregnancy because of the danger of miscarriage. Years ago, when travel may have meant separation from good medical facilities, the advice could have been warranted. Today, if your pregnancy is normal, there is no reason not to travel, especially before the last month. Fetuses aren't so delicate that they can be harmed by a bumpy plane trip or long hours of driving; if problems arise, medical help is almost always nearby.

Some ways pregnant women make extended traveling more comfortable are to schedule vacations for the middle trimester when discomforts usually disappear; get rooms with private baths when abroad, even if they wouldn't ordinarily; plan sightseeing around nap times; avoid over-the-counter drugs abroad, where marketing standards may be unfamiliar. Extended domestic travel is usually very easy because of the familiarity of facilities, food, and lodging. If you don't know a physician in the area where you are traveling, you can always go to a hospital emergency room.

Tips for car travel

While not harmful, long car trips can often be uncomfortable. The seat belt, confinement, and bucket seats make traveling awkward. To minimize discomforts:

• Bring a Thermos of juice, as well as cheese, fruit, and sandwiches.

• Stop every sixty minutes—at a minimum—for five to ten minutes. Get out of the car and walk, exercise, or stretch. While in the car, periodically press the small of your back into the back of the car seat to relieve lower-back tightness.

• If you are nauseated, it sometimes helps to *drive* rather than remain a passenger.

• Mark out rest-room stops before you start your trip, so that you'll know when you *must* stop and when you can afford to pass one up. A motor club can help you here.

• Bring a pair of gym shoes or slippers for the car. Long periods of sitting can cause your feet to swell, and it's definitely a relief to switch to soft, expandable shoes. Also, don't sit with legs crossed; this position hinders circulation.

• Be aware, if you are taking turns driving, that you will tire more quickly when pregnant, even if you're only sitting and driving. When tired, you may be more accident prone.

• Bring a pillow, and a blanket if necessary, so that you can lie on your left side in the back seat. This will minimize edema and pelvic congestion. Take along a rolled-up towel to place in the small of your back for support while sitting.

• One researcher (Dr. C. D. Matthews), studying the value of seat belts for pregnant women, came to these conclusions: (1) if you do *not* wear a restraint system, you run a greater risk of damaging your uterus and the fetus in an accident than if you wear one (this should reassure pregnant women who worry that seat belts can actually damage the baby); (2) tests on baboons showed a shoulder anchor plus a lap belt greatly enhanced the chances for fetal survival in an accident; (3) for greatest fetal safety in an accident, wear the *whole* safety system: harness and belt. Keep the belt tight and low (across the thighs, not the abdomen), and place a cushion between the abdomen and the seat belt.

Air travel

Traveling by air is much easier than traveling by car. However, there are several myths surrounding plane travel and pregnancy. Some of them are:

1. *Cabin pressurization can harm the fetus.* There has never been any evidence linking flying to fetal problems. Decades ago, when pregnant women flew in planes far less well pressurized than now, neither they nor their babies experienced any difficulties.

2. *If you should need oxygen because of decompression, the fetus may be damaged.* Because this occurrence is so rare, no statistics are available on how decompression affects the fetus. According to Robert L. Wick, Jr., M.D., medical director of American Airlines, "The use of oxygen during a decompression would not present a danger to either mother or fetus. However, the failure to use oxygen would represent a serious omission on the part of the mother and would represent the same risk as it would to any passenger."

3. *You can be stopped from boarding the plane if you appear to be close to delivery.* Years ago, some airlines required a note from the obstetrician of a woman who was flying during her last month of pregnancy. The International Air Transport Association recommends that no expectant mother be allowed on a plane within seven days of her expected delivery date. Rules like these are usually impossible to enforce, and unnecessary, too, because women are generally ca-

pable of deciding for themselves, after talking to their physicians, whether they should travel. The likelihood of anyone detaining you during boarding is remote unless you're visibly ill or in labor.

A woman having trouble with her pregnancy may want to talk to her physician about the advisability of flying. Her doctor can consult with the various airline medical departments for more information.

Because domestic air travel is so fast and comfortable, there isn't too much you can do to enhance it. A few suggestions, though:

• Get tickets in advance by mail to avoid lines at ticket counters.

• Consider ordering a special vegetarian meal if you can't eat meat.

• To keep comfortable, ask for pillows and put one in the small of your back. Those little airline pillows are the perfect size for support of the lumbar spine. If the seat belt is uncomfortable, put a pillow between it and your abdomen.

• Ask for a seat near the restroom (often, however, that will also be in the smoking section). Be sure to get an aisle seat if you're in your last trimester. Finally, you may want to try getting a bulkhead seat (behind the partition). It provides a bit more legroom.

• Don't panic if you go into labor on the plane. First labors average fourteen hours, and subsequent labors average eight hours. Most continental flights take four hours or less, and no matter where you are, the pilot can make an emergency landing in about thirty minutes. Very soon thereafter, you can be in a hospital.

• Very long flights are not comfortable, and probably not advisable, during the last month of pregnancy. It helps to walk around, flex and extend your extremities, roll your shoulders, avoid alcohol, and eat lightly. Bring a pair of gym shoes or slippers and wear comfortable, loose-fitting clothes.

Traveling abroad

If you are going abroad, particularly if you are headed for underdeveloped nations, various vaccinations may be required or desirable to guard against such diseases as cholera, smallpox, yellow fever, tetanus, and typhoid. Unfortunately, nobody knows the effect of many immunizations on unborn children. It is often advisable to forgo travel rather than be vaccinated if you are pregnant. If you think you *may* be pregnant, tell the physician who is going to immunize you. If you *know* you are pregnant, but still have to travel to a country where vaccination is required or desirable, talk first with your obstetrician.

The following information on diseases is from bulletins published by the American College of Obstetricians and Gynecologists and the U.S. Public Health Service:

• *Typhoid.* Prevalent in many countries of Africa, Asia, Central and South America. How the disease affects the fetus isn't known, but there is a high mortality among adults. While there is no confirmed risk to the fetus from the vaccine, it is "not recommended during pregnancy" by the U.S. Public Health Service.

• *Yellow fever.* Prevalent in parts of Africa and South America. The effects of the vaccine on the fetus are unknown, but the ACOG bulletin notes that it is better to postpone a trip than take the vaccine.

• *Cholera.* The risk of contracting cholera is low. The U.S. Public Health Service says that "immunization is not routinely recommended for travelers to countries not requiring vaccination as a condition for entry." The effects of the vaccine on the fetus are unknown.

• *Smallpox.* Considered eradicated, but has appeared recently in Ethiopia. A pregnant woman should *not* take this vaccine; the U.S. Public Health Service lists pregnancy as a contraindication.

• *Tetanus.* Everyone—whether traveling or staying at home— should have an up-to-date immunity to tetanus because the deadly tetanus organism is found all over the world. Booster injections are good for up to ten years; the ACOG bulletin states: "Updating of immune status should be part of antepartum care."

• *Poliomyelitis.* Persons traveling to underdeveloped areas may be exposed to poliomyelitis. The U.S. Public Health Service recommends either a booster dose or a primary immunization. There is no confirmed risk to the fetus from the vaccine.

Patients who wish to travel must do a balancing act. Is the risk of disease greater than the unknown and unconfirmed hazards to the fetus caused by the vaccine? The question is a difficult one to answer; and if the travel involved is for pleasure, it would seem prudent to postpone trips to areas where certain diseases are prevalent. The ACOG bulletin sums it up: "During pregnancy it is preferable, if possible, to reduce exposure rather than vaccinate when live virus vaccines are involved. A pregnant woman can avoid certain diseases by not entering areas endemic for those diseases."

Sports and exercise

Americans are cautious about pregnancy; we're amazed when we see an expectant mother horseback-riding or running a marathon. Yet, increasingly, women are active in sports before pregnancy and want to continue their interests while pregnant. Is this activity beneficial or harmful? Nobody really knows about most sports because few studies have been done.

We know that pregnancy increases cardiovascular output, oxygen consumption, and fatigue; and we know how it changes weight, balance, and hormone levels, and how the pelvic and sacroiliac joints relax. How will these factors relate to your activities? To start with:

1. Check with your physician about the sport you wish to pursue.

2. While you exercise, pay careful attention to your body for signs of fatigue, strain, or discomfort.

Athletes pursuing competitive sports have special needs. They should consult a physician familiar with sports medicine. In general, the following statements are true about sports during pregnancy:

• Some health-care professionals believe that risks to the fetus from active sports are greatest during the first trimester and that activity should be *limited* then. Others, like Dr. James A. Nicholas of the Institute of Sports Medicine and Athletic Trauma, believe: "In early pregnancy, most sports can be continued as usual. After the fifth month there is a viable fetus and though the evidence is scant, it would appear advisable for the mother to avoid skiing and contact sports." The debate seems to offer no sure answer for everyone. Diver Juno Irwin and skier Andrea Mead Lawrence both won Olympic medals in their first trimesters; others have played softball and run marathons during their last.

• The sports you do undertake during pregnancy should be the same ones you participated in before you were pregnant.

• Pregnant athletes are more likely to experience strains because of already strained joints. Therefore, a good warm-up before activity is essential. Fifteen minutes of easy stretching or simple walking helps send blood to muscles and helps avoid stiffness and injury.-

• You must tune into your body closely to determine its limits. First, honestly assess yourself in the following areas: balance, coordination, speed, agility, endurance, and strength. Next, analyze the sports you like best, and you'll get an idea of which you'll be most comfortable with. Judging your limits must continue while you are active. Stop when you are tired. It will take you much longer to get your energy back than it did before you were pregnant.

• What can exercise do *for* you? Improve your muscle tone and circulation and minimize fatigue and back pain. Some studies indicate that athletic women have less painful labors, easier deliveries, and fewer cesareans. But other researchers believe that a high degree of physical fitness has no effect on ease or length of birth, or may make delivery more difficult because of strong, well-developed perineal muscles. There is some evidence that athletic women enjoy a speedier postpartum recovery.

• Because breasts enlarge during pregnancy, you may be more comfortable wearing a bra while running, playing tennis or other competitive sports, or exercising.

Which sports?

• *Tennis.* Good if you can moderate your game somewhat. Sharp twists and sudden stops can strain pelvic ligaments, especially during the last trimester; also, some serves that require a deeply arched back should be abandoned temporarily. To avoid muscle problems, keep knees loose and bent. Transfer weight smoothly from foot to foot. If the day is hot, wear a hat and watch for signs of heat exhaustion (fatigue, headache, dizziness), which may come on faster than usual. Also, consider playing doubles, which may be less strenuous when you're pregnant.

• *Racquetball.* Observe the same precautions as above. Those, however, who play in air-conditioned clubs must be careful that their bodies don't cool down too fast (muscle aches may result, and they're particularly hard to dispel during pregnancy). Bring along a warm-up jacket and put it on after each match. Stay bundled after you shower until the room no longer feels cool. Also, the small court and fast-moving ball may make racquetball hazardous in the later months.

• *Walking.* Often called the best exercise for an expectant mother, walking tones all the muscles and is less tiring than other activities. It promotes good circulation, better posture, and general body conditioning.

• *Running.* Researchers are just now looking into the effects on pregnancy of running. Some tests following individuals or small selected groups of pregnant women runners seem to indicate no problems, but because of individual differences, each woman should check with her physician.

Runner and physician Dr. Joan Ullyot says in her excellent book *Women's Running* that running is fine during pregnancy as long as you do what you're accustomed to and work comfortably. To check, take the talk test. If you can chat comfortably to your partner or yourself, you're not overdoing it.

Because you tire more easily when pregnant and can't bounce back quickly after working out, you may want to modify your running routine during the early and late months. For example, alternate running with walking, or reduce running time by a quarter. Running every other day may make a difference because you allow yourself recovery time. On hot days, drink lots of fluids and wear a hat. Above all, don't push yourself. Even military guidelines say it's too hot to run when the temperature goes above 85° F. Other things to avoid: racing, hard surfaces, large daily increases in mileage, marathons if they are new to you, stopping without a warm-up jacket available. Do read running magazines, which often feature articles on pregnancy.

• *Swimming.* Another top-notch sport during pregnancy. Because it's not competitive or aggressive, swimming can be soothing and relaxing. The water supports your weight (relieving pelvic ligaments), while stroking and kicking develop body tone, stretch muscles, and increase endurance. The breast- and sidestroke are generally less strenuous than the front crawl or backstroke. No matter which stroke you use, you may want to rest every few lengths, and certainly stop if you experience abdominal discomfort or leg cramps. Also, caution is called for around slippery pool decks.

• *Bicycle riding.* An excellent sport during pregnancy, although balance may be difficult during the last months. (A stationary bicycle is a good idea if you want only the exercise, because there is less risk of falling.) Don't add to the problem by seating a child on your bike. To check balance, see how well you can bike along a straight line. If your bike is wobbling, try keeping your body straighter or shift to a lower gear. Backache and leg cramps are sometimes problems. Backache can be relieved by changing where and how you grip the handlebars; leg cramps will be less of a problem if you can intermittently flex and rotate feet and wiggle toes while riding. Finally, drink plenty of fluids on windy days. You may be perspiring profusely and not realize it because of rapid evaporation.

• *Backpacking.* This isn't a good time to hike with a twenty-five- or thirty-pound load on your back—the last thing you need is more strain on those muscles. In addition, the frame backpack with its hip strap may really throw off your balance because it switches the center of gravity from the hips to the shoulders. Add to these problems swollen feet, trailless terrain that requires sure footing, and you've got an activity that is extremely difficult for pregnant women. As a variant, pack a soft rucksack and take a day hike along a trail. You can still cook out, gobble goodies, and enjoy the outdoors without risking strain. If you need to purify water, go ahead. Halazone tablets are probably safe to use during pregnancy, and, of course, so is boiled water.

• *Golf.* This may be good during the early months; after all, nine holes of golf may equal two miles of walking. However, in later months, the twisting may put quite a strain on pelvic ligaments. That same twisting, plus bending, may make *bowling* difficult, too.

• *To be avoided: surfing, waterskiing, and swimming in pounding surf* (in each, a fall may force water up the vagina); *snow skiing* during the second half of pregnancy (too great a chance of a dangerous fall); *vigorous gymnastics* (some activities like balance beam and uneven parallel bars present a risk of falling); *hang gliding; skydiving; skin diving* (after the second trimester).

Two important exercises

If there's no athletic activity that you've been pursuing, but you still want to be in good condition during pregnancy, there are a number of excellent exercises that, when organized, can form a daily routine. Even women who run or swim every day should follow an exercise program designed for expectant mothers. Elizabeth

Noble's *Essential Exercises for the Childbearing Year* contains such a program and is a gem of a book—clear and precise. Meanwhile, two exercises that you'll hear about often and are musts while pregnant:

• *Kegel exercise.* Exercises the pelvic floor; develops support for uterus and all pelvic organs; and relieves pelvic congestion. To do the exercise, alternately contract and release the muscles of the pelvic floor (to become familiar with the sensation, try stopping and starting the flow of urine).

• *Pelvic rock.* Relieves backache and tightens abdominal muscles. While lying on your back with knees bent and feet on floor, press the small of the back into the floor. You should feel the whole pelvic region "tilting" back. Once you get a feel for the movement, you can do this exercise while standing, lying on your side, or on hands and knees (in which case it is called the "angry cat" because of the rounded shape of the back).

Sleeping

Most women find that they need more sleep while pregnant, and they get it either by napping or by going to bed earlier. No matter how busy you are, *don't deny yourself the extra sleep,* for it is a fundamental need now. You'll do yourself a great disservice if you go into labor ill rested.

Problems with sleeping

During pregnancy, certain conditions, such as nausea and the need to urinate in the middle of the night, conspire to deny you sleep. Other difficulties include:

• *The baby's kicking.* Some researchers theorize that the baby is active when you are at rest precisely because there is no movement to lull it to sleep. Others believe that being awake at night is just part of some babies' cycles. You can try changing positions or rocking on hands and knees in bed to calm the baby. Some women swear that stroking and singing to the abdomen helps.

• *Indigestion.* Aside from the tips on page 64, allow yourself at least one and a half hours between your last meal and your bedtime. This will give your digestive system a chance to absorb the food.

•*Stuffy nose.* Sleep on an extra pillow if it makes breathing easier (this often relieves nausea, too). Sometimes a vaporizer will help if your mucous membranes are dry and irritated.

•*Positioning.* It's hard to find a comfortable sleeping position, especially during the last month. Rearrangement of pillows and close attention to the parts of your body susceptible to strain are important. The *supine,* or back, position is generally not comfortable because it shifts the uterus onto the large veins, obstructing blood flow. While supine, you may feel all the symptoms of the resulting low blood pressure: dizziness, nausea, palpitations. If so, lying on your side will bring immediate relief. If you have no problem sleeping on your back and really prefer that position, a small pillow under the small of your back and one beneath your knees will reduce strain. As long as you have no adverse symptoms, it's safe to sleep in this position.

Lying on your stomach may also be uncomfortable during later months. There is, however, no danger to the baby in this position. Lying on your side, legs spread comfortably as if running, may be the easiest sleeping position. A small pillow or folded towel under your lower abdomen and a long pillow against your back will provide support. If you keep one leg atop the other, a pillow between them will be comfortable.

•*Sleeping conditions.* Air conditioning is a must in the summer for comfortable sleeping if you are in your last month or two. In the winter, hot chocolate may seem enticing before bed, but be prepared to pay the price when you have to urinate at 3:00 A.M.

•*Relaxing.* Relaxation techniques are important: deep breathing, mentally loosening and letting go of all tenseness in every part of the body; yoga; Lamaze techniques. These are worthwhile to practice during the day, too.

Housework and family care

Housework is hard work. Constant bending, lifting, and carrying can strain the ligaments of the back and pelvis. If you reserve chores for the evening, you may have to do them in a fatigued state and lose an opportunity to rest. Ideals about what your house should look like conflict with what you actually have the time and ability to accomplish if your strength has been diminished by pregnancy.

Family care is more rewarding than housecleaning, yet there are difficulties associated with it, too. Lifting and running after young children, constant exposure to colds and sicknesses, minimal time to relax or rest, and more time devoted to cleaning and straightening—all can cause fatigue or a sense of being drained and exhausted. If you have young children and your energy is limited because of your pregnancy, you may feel divided and unsure about how to allot your time.

Above all, if fatigue or stress is a problem, cut out nonessential activities and, if you can afford it, hire help. You have to decide for yourself which activities to omit, but do force a change if it gives you more time to rest. Other tips:

• Preserve your back. Pregnancy causes the joints in the lower back to relax, so that bending can strain your muscles. Keep your back straight; squat to pick up both light and heavy objects (pins, books, groceries, children); and hold onto something for balance, if necessary.

• Bending over dishes, groceries, automatic dryers, and dishwashers can also hurt your back. If you can't *raise* the object, *squat* to work at it.

• Reaching high can strain the small of the back, so be sure to use a stool or stepladder when you need something from the top shelf.

• Elevated noise levels can cause a rise in blood pressure, increased heart rate, irritability, tension, and anxiety. When you're fatigued and particularly vulnerable to these stresses, minimize the use of the vacuum cleaner, blender, food mixer, dishwasher, and hair dryer.

• Teach little children to maneuver for themselves—to crawl into car seats and strollers (strap them in, of course), to stand on chairs to be lifted, to put on their own coats, and to pick up toys. Any kind of twisting you do to carry little ones, such as holding them on the hip, can hurt pelvic joints.

• Work on all fours when feasible.

• Gardeners should work on hands and knees or in a tailor position, intermittently rolling the shoulders and rotating the head to avoid stiffness. Keep tools, bags, and fertilizer close to avoid constant rising and dropping down. Handle tools such as power mowers with care, remembering that your balance and footing may be less sure than before. Always wear protective clothing and use a sunscreen for extended work outdoors. Gardeners should also wear gloves to protect them from soil microorganisms that transmit toxoplasmosis (see page 47).

• Keep stair-climbing (which means carrying your weight against gravity) to a minimum. If you live in a two-story residence, keep two sets of cleaning materials, diapers, scissors, pencils, paper, for both floors. Store all outerwear, such as sweaters, gloves, hats, boots, and outdoor sports equipment, downstairs.

• If you must stand in lines while shopping, keep feet and legs moving; sway and rock to keep from fainting—a relatively common problem that accompanies decreased circulation.

Hazards in the home

It is not enough to be vigilant about sources of fatigue and physical hazards in the home. You should be aware of possible chemical hazards, too. Some twenty-five thousand new chemical compounds are developed every year. They may appear in oven cleaners and aerosols, in laundering aids and furniture polish, in paints and insecticides. We breathe them, touch them, and in some cases eat them.

Appropriate tests for teratogenicity (damage to the fetus) are not run on these chemicals because such tests are not required by law. Nobody knows which of these substances, once inside the mother's body, can cross the placenta and affect the fetus. Worse, we do not know which compounds can deform or abort fetuses, and which can induce cancer when that fetus grows to adulthood.

The picture is even more complex. Two or more harmless compounds, when ingested together, may have lethal results for an organism. One benign compound, in the presence of heat from, say, a radiator or stove, may change to a toxic by-product. Some toxic chemicals take decades to work their damage. Some experts estimate that 2 to 3 percent of all congenital malformations can be attributed to drugs or to toxic chemicals in the environment. The combinations of environmental and genetic effects may cause many more.

Recently, an environmental advocate, commenting on the variety of toxic chemicals present in our homes, exclaimed that no chemist would dare handle these substances as haphazardly as does the average consumer. We fail to read warning labels, wear protective clothing, masks, and goggles, follow directions. If so many of our household cleaning and convenience items can cause rashes, dizziness, allergy, dangerous fumes, and burns, can we be sure that when we inhale them they will have no effect on our unborn children? Can we be certain that chemicals considered non-toxic for adults are safe for fetuses, whose tissues and organs are more likely to be damaged because they are undergoing rapid growth?

The answer is that we cannot. And we cannot turn for solutions to our physicians, who generally are not well schooled in environmental health. Nor can we depend on manufacturers or the government, because a product's appearance on the market is not a guarantee of safety. It is up to each of us to exercise special caution during pregnancy, temporarily limiting or abandoning those activities that place us in contact with questionable substances.

Being careful

• Use all household cleaners, particularly volatile or fume-producing ones, in well-ventilated rooms. Open windows and doors before you spray, pour, or apply cleaners. This is particularly important in small, enclosed areas like closets and bathrooms.

• Cut down on aerosol use. Every aerosol contains an active ingredient (deodorant, defogger, cleaner, and so on) and a propellant packed under pressure. Unlike pump sprays and liquids, the aerosol product (propellant plus ingredient) comes out in extremely small droplets that can burrow their way deep into the respiratory tract and get quickly absorbed into the bloodstream and reach the placenta. Several studies link aerosol use not only to birth defects in test animals but to cardiac and respiratory problems, liver damage, nausea, and cancer. When you do use aerosols, provide good ventilation. If you use any of the following in aerosol form, consider substituting the nonaerosol counterpart: air fresheners; window, counter, tile, and oven cleaners; spot removers; deodorants; hair sprays; water repellants for shoes and boots; disinfectants; furniture polish.

• Dry-cleaning solvents give off dangerous fumes. Carbon tetrachloride, on the market for years, was removed because of its high toxicity, but many other dangerous cleaning chemicals are still commonly used, and nobody has tested them for fetal toxicity. When using coin-operated dry-cleaning machines, be careful not to inhale fumes, and open windows if you can. After the machine stops, open the door and move away to allow the fumes to dissipate.

• If you plan to have an exterminator in your house or apartment, leave the premises during the work and try not to return for several hours. When you do, open the windows and doors to get rid of the fumes.

• Extreme caution must be taken when using insecticides, rodenticides, herbicides, and defoliants. By and large, these materials have not been tested for teratogenicity, but—to be safe—assume that any chemical lethal to insects can be harmful to us. Can insecticides and the like reach the fetus? One study several years ago detected DDT in the cord blood of newborn infants.

There isn't much we can do about the extremely potent agricultural pesticides sprayed on crops, such as the chlorinated hydrocarbons, including aldrin, endrin, dieldrin, and many more (heptachlor, now banned, had been detected in the organs of stillborn infants). These linger in the environment and are detectable in virtually all animal tissue. We should, of course, thoroughly scrub all fruits and vegetables (although many of these toxic substances are found in the meat we consume). In our own gardens we should minimize or omit the use of pesticides. If you read the labels, you'll find such warnings as "Keep away from children and pets," "Wear waterproof gloves, face shield, and goggles when applying," and "This product is toxic to fish and wildlife." Don't assume the product cannot harm the fetus—most insecticides have not been tested for this danger. Presume that any product unsafe for children is even less safe for unborn children. Treat pesticides as you would medicines and drugs. Inside the house, check all pesticides—not only aerosol, but solid or continuous-release types, too. Use powdered silica gel, for instance, to take care of insects indoors; it is safer for human health. Materials not safe for use in infants' rooms, children's rooms, playrooms, or hospital rooms are probably not safe around pregnant women, either.

And it should be noted that pesticides can harm the reproductive system of men, too, causing abnormalities and even abortion of the fertilized egg.

About refinishing that crib . . .

During pregnancy, while getting things ready for the baby, many women tackle major carpentry and painting projects. They may wallpaper, paint, and sand, or strip and refinish cribs, cradles, dressers, woodwork, floors, dressing tables, and toys. In so doing, they breathe in a variety of vapors, fumes, and dusts, and contact many chemicals that may be hazardous not only to their health but to their baby's as well.

Recently, attention has been given to the safety of artists' tools, chemicals, and environments. Unfortunately, there is little known about the hazards of these materials to pregnant women and their babies. It is up to each individual working with volatile chemicals, dyes, metals, dusts, and gases to exercise caution. We should all be careful about the tasks we assign ourselves; perhaps our plans for redecorating or remodeling should be kept to a minimum or be carried out by someone else.

Much of the following information and advice comes from a recently published guide for artists, *Safe Practices in the Arts and Crafts: A Studio Guide,* by Gail Coningsby Barazani:

• "Pregnant women should not work with solvents or substances containing solvents, ever." These include stripping compounds, paint and varnish removers, paint and lacquer cleaners, stains, and some paints and varnishes. Some of the chemicals to look out for and avoid while pregnant: aromatic hydrocarbons, benzene (benzol), toluene, xylene (xylol), dimethyl benzene, cumene, styrene, methylene chloride, ethylene dichloride, trichloroethylene, alcohol (aliphatic and aromatic amyl, butyl), methanol, acetone, aldehydes, formaldehyde. Some are known to be dangerous to the fetus; others may cause changes in the mother's respiratory, cardiovascular, or nervous system, which could indirectly harm the unborn child.

• If you *must* work with a volatile solvent (a solvent that gives off vapors), follow these precautions:

1. Thoroughly ventilate the room by opening windows, doors, and exhausts. Don't recycle vapor-laden air through the air conditioner.

2. Wear protective clothing, including gloves.

3. Wear a respirator, not a disposable filter mask. The respirator should say it is approved by NIOSH (National Institute of Occupational Safety and Health) or MESA (Mining and Engineers Safety Administration). Many respirators use interchangeable cartridges. To obtain the appropriate respirator and cartridges, check the Yellow Pages for safety supply companies.

4. Do not eat, drink, or smoke in the work area.

5. Discard rags that release solvents into the air.

6. Vaporization of solvents occurs quickly when the weather is warm. Keep the room temperature below 70° F. if possible.

7. Purchase solvents labeled "pure." Never leave solvents uncovered.

• Latex paints are probably the safest to work with, but *exterior* paints often contain a mercury fungicide, and mercury compounds are extremely hazardous to unborn children. When cleaning your tools, don't leave brushes standing in open jars of solvent.

• Dusts and fumes of metallic compounds—in particular, lead, cadmium, and mercury—are especially hazardous to the fetus. If you are stripping paint that may be more than twenty years old, it may contain lead. Wear a respirator—or, better yet, leave the job to someone else.

• Be sure patching compounds are labeled "asbestos-free." Asbestos may be carcinogenic to the fetus as well as to the mother.

• Avoid working in the kitchen, where food can be contaminated. And don't use eating utensils for your art projects.

If you have any questions about materials you want to work with or procedures that may be hazardous, write to the Art Hazards Information Center, 5 Beekman Street, New York, NY 10038. Telephone: 212-227-6220.

Health care

Unless your physician specializes in family practice, health care can be bewildering when you are pregnant. In this era of medical specialization, your treatments and checkups may be fragmented among, for example, an obstetrician, an internist, a urologist, and a dermatologist. Many families use the nearest hospital emergency room as a primary-care center, and if you have unusual problems, you may be in the care of still other specialists. So it's hard to know, when you are feeling ill, whom to see.

During pregnancy, you may delay seeing a physician simply because you don't know whom to call. When you are taking care of yourself, *never self-medicate.* No drug is absolutely safe when you're pregnant. Aspirin, long thought to produce birth defects in the human fetus, has been proved to cause malformations in the embryos of laboratory animals. Some studies have shown that a greater percentage of mothers with malformed infants took aspirin than did mothers of normal babies. If you are tempted to try some antibiotics you have in the medicine cabinet—*don't.* Some are suspected teratogens. Sedatives, antidepressants, and over-the-counter remedies all may be dangerous to the developing fetus. *Do not self-medicate.*

How, then, do you handle sickness? If it's a cold, just keep warm and rested, and try to relieve your symptoms without medication: with a vaporizer, rest, and liquids. Nasal sprays, which can elevate blood pressure, should be avoided. A thousand milligrams of vitamin C (a common dose for cold sufferers) is probably all right—the vitamin is water-soluble and easily excreted. If you have a fever, call your physician.

For a headache, you can take Tylenol after the first twelve weeks of pregnancy. During the first trimester, you might get headache relief with a cold washcloth, quiet, and rest.

There's no truth to the myth that pregnant women have more resistance to disease. Acute upper respiratory infections, for example, may even be worse during pregnancy.

Many times when pregnant women know there's a need to consult about an illness, they wonder which of their physicians to call. If you are seeing a specialist about a particular problem and you suddenly develop a physical ailment related to it, call that specialist first. Your obstetrician and specialist may have already established contact concerning your case. If not, be sure to tell the specialist that you are or may be pregnant. If medicine, X rays, or any course of treatment is prescribed, say that you would like to check first with your obstetrician before undertaking the treatment.

Don't be afraid of offending your physician, but contact your obstetrician quickly. It is likely (but not certain) that an obstetrician will be more familiar with teratogenic or abortifacient (abortion-inducing) substances than a physician in another field. If you don't yet have an obstetrician, you might ask a pediatrician's opinion of recommended medication. Pediatricians are also familiar with fetal health.

If you find yourself with a sore throat, flu, diarrhea, swollen glands, fever, or any other minor ailment that seems completely unrelated to your reproductive system or pregnancy, call your obstetrician, anyway. For many women, the obstetrician-gynecologist is the primary health care giver, and s/he is accustomed to calls about a variety of health matters. A good obstetrician should be consulted about, or be the one to prescribe, any medication a pregnant woman takes.

Don't be afraid to ask about any medications prescribed. If possible, obtain a library copy of the *Physicians' Desk Reference* so that you can see for yourself the possible side effects and contraindications of what's been prescribed for you. Then take your medication as directed for as long as directed.

Treat yourself considerately. The cumulative effects of pregnancy and illness can be debilitating. If you are accustomed to bouncing back from illness quickly, you may be surprised when your recovery is slowed. It helps to pay careful attention to bedrest and diet, and to ease back into your usual activities.

Eye care

If parts of your body are retaining fluid, as often happens during pregnancy, your eyes may, too, and the shape of your eyeball will be affected. Eyeglass wearers may not notice the change, but contact-lens wearers (especially those who have hard lenses) may suddenly feel discomfort—enough to return to wearing glasses. Just remember that this condition is temporary and eye shape will return to normal after delivery.

Oral hygiene and teeth care

During pregnancy there is an increase in estrogen and progesterone production. In the same way these hormones cause congestion in the uterus, they cause congestion and swelling of gums. If teeth and gums are not carefully cleaned during pregnancy, irritation, bleeding, and inflammation of the gums will result. Some women even develop a bit of extra inflamed tissue on their gums. This painless growth often disappears after delivery. (If not, it must be removed.)

Brushing your teeth after every meal and flossing are good practices for everyone; they are particularly important for pregnant women. Any plaque on the teeth is an irritant. It's wise to visit a dentist for a checkup early in pregnancy to have your teeth cleaned.

Another way to keep your teeth healthy is to eat a balanced diet. This, combined with good oral hygiene, will minimize caries. Tooth decay is not accelerated by pregnancy. Nor is it true that a baby can drain calcium from the mother's teeth. In cases of extreme calcium deficiency, the calcium for the fetus comes from the mother's bones.

Dental X rays

Many women are reluctant to visit a dentist during pregnancy because they worry about the danger of X rays taken during checkups. Certainly you must always let your dentist know that you are, or think you are, pregnant. This may affect the course of treatment. Yet the question remains: Should you permit dental X rays during pregnancy?

Aiming an X-ray beam directly at a fetus can be hazardous if the X-ray dose is high. A fetus, whose tissues are in a state of rapid growth, is much more likely to experience radiation damage—at any stage of its development—than an adult. Dental X rays, however, do not significantly affect your reproductive organs because they are aimed at the mouth. In a recent symposium, Dr. Ray W. Alcox noted that dental X-ray exposure to reproductive organs is minimal. He said ". . . the amount of scatter radiation to the gonadal area from a full mouth survey approximates that from a day's normal background radiation [that is, from the sun's rays]." If your dentist's equipment is modern and in good working order (the dentist uses high-speed film, a properly collimated and filtrated beam, and an open-ended, properly shielded cone), and you wear a lead apron, dental X rays should be safe. Nevertheless, many practitioners come down on the side of caution and will do no X rays at all on pregnant women.

Elective dental treatment (as opposed to regular checkups or treatment for nondelayable problems) is best postponed, if possible, until after delivery, or done in the second trimester when the risk of abortion is past and before the fetus is so large that lying in a dental chair can cause the patient to feel faint. Some general anesthetics may cause birth defects early in pregnancy. Local anesthesia should be used instead.

A dental emergency may require drugs, but these should be prescribed very carefully. You might ask that your dentist consult with your obstetrician. Some antibiotics (such as tetracycline) and aspirin are suspected of causing birth defects. The possible hazards of many other drugs are not known.

Besides protecting your teeth, you can also protect your *baby's* teeth, prenatally, through proper diet. Being aware of nutrition is important early in pregnancy, as tooth development actually begins seven to eight weeks after fertilization. Many viral infections (such as rubella) and even fever in the mother can affect the size, shape, and enamel of the baby's teeth. Antibiotics such as Achromycin, Panmycin, Aureomycin, and Terramycin, taken during pregnancy, can actually stain the baby's teeth gray, orange, or yellow. Nevertheless, eating well and avoiding drugs is about all you can do to ensure healthy teeth for your child. For unless you are grossly undernourished, teeth develop and grow as they were patterned to genetically.

After hours

Being pregnant doesn't mean cutting out your social life. For many women, though, particularly in the last trimester, it means adapting your usual activities for greater comfort.

• **Restaurants.** If a restaurant is popular and there's apt to be a long wait that would make you tired, phone ahead. Ask if there is seating in an anteroom or at a bar. If not, explain that you cannot stand for long periods and ask if they can pinpoint a seating time. Be aware, also, that waiting in a foyer can mean enduring hot, stuffy, smoky surroundings. Women who have been experiencing nausea should probably avoid unfamiliar cuisines.

• **Theaters.** Often, seat backs are too short, legroom is nonexistent, armrests are uncomfortable—and that's when you're not pregnant. When you're in your ninth month and will be sitting through a movie or play, try to get an aisle seat so that you can stretch your legs. Periodically pushing the small of your back into the back of the chair (the pelvic rock) will release tension and ease backache.

• **Cocktail parties.** Avoid alcohol. Eat at the beginning of the party so that you have time to digest food before going to sleep at night. Leave early if you find it uncomfortable to stand in smoky, stuffy rooms.

• **Stadium games.** Avoid bleacher seats if they mean scaling the heights late in pregnancy; if your back aches, the lack of seat backs will be especially uncomfortable. Climbing lots of stairs may leave you short of breath and with aching legs. At all times, minimize exposure to the sun by wearing protective clothing and sunscreen preparations, and by sitting in shaded areas. Finally, come early and leave late to avoid jostling crowds.

CHAPTER TWELVE
How to Look Great

Most American men and women spend considerable time and money on grooming and cosmetics. Perhaps because of innate vanity or advertising indoctrination, most of us want to look attractive and will often go to great lengths to ensure this result. For pregnant women, however, the physical, emotional, and psychological changes of their condition often take precedence over such concerns as hair and skin care.

Yet pregnancy may require that you devote *more* time to grooming. Many women report that they feel better if they pay extra attention to their makeup and hair. Some women work harder at their face and hair simply to compensate for the feeling of being less attractive. For whatever reason, careful grooming should be a part of an expectant mother's life, just as it is for every other woman.

Pregnancy itself presents unique makeup problems. Recently, some cosmetics companies have become more aware of these specific needs. Lady Madonna Manufacturing Company, for example, now markets a line of skin and hair products geared especially for pregnant women. (Of course, you needn't buy cosmetics especially formulated for pregnant women.)

Changes in hair

Some women are startled by excessive thinning or falling out of hair during pregnancy. After delivery, some new mothers may even find themselves with bald patches. Losing about a hundred hairs a day is a normal phenomenon, but pregnancy often increases that number, to the dismay of women who may feel this is just another indication of an upset in their bodily systems. Experts have a variety of opinions on the reason for such hair loss: lack of sufficient iron or certain vitamins; inadequate diet; production of HCG or other hormones that inhibit hair growth; stress; even the body's need to focus its energies on more crucial processes than hair growth.

Unfortunately, there do not seem to be any effective ways of stopping hair loss or stimulating hair growth during pregnancy, except to wait for the body to return to its nonpregnant state. Since the substances in your blood can help hair to grow and flourish, a good diet, including sufficient vitamins and minerals, may retard its loss. Generally, thinning hair should be treated with care. Wash your hair regularly with a mild shampoo and use a cream rinse or conditioner.

Balsam and protein conditioners and shampoos will add fullness to your hair by actually coating the strands. The less you manipulate it, though, the better. Always use a soft-bristled brush and a wide-toothed comb. A fingertip massage of the scalp *may* help hair growth and health, though experts disagree as to the effectiveness of this treatment. A simple-to-care-for hairstyle will minimize the amount of handling your hair must have to look its best. If your style requires frequent blow-drying or setting with a curling iron or electric rollers to make it work, you'll run the risk of losing even more hair. Even if you have healthy hair, but continually pull it into a ponytail or cornrows, you may get a type of hair loss known as traction alopecia.

Besides an easy-to-manage style (and this may mean a shorter cut), you might want to consider a wig or hairpiece. Take time to have the wig fitted correctly. See that you're thoroughly comfortable in it, and that the wig is compatible with your facial coloring. Since pregnant women often perspire more, it's best not to wear the wig more than a few hours at a time. The increased perspiration from prolonged wear may cause itching and aggravate dandruff. According to some beauty specialists, excessive wear may even retard hair growth.

Thinning hair during pregnancy should not be further stressed by permanent hair coloring, waving, and straightening treatments, which cause major changes in even the healthiest hair. Such treatments can have devastating effects on hair that's not in its best condition.

Hair coloring

Many women believe coloring their hair makes it more attractive or gives them a needed psychological boost. But if you're pregnant you may want to consider a few other matters before you begin or continue to color your hair.

The three major types of hair coloring are: (1) temporary; (2) semipermanent; and (3) permanent.

Temporary colors damage hair very little, and so are suitable for expectant mothers with dry, thinning, or weakened hair. Nevertheless, the color usually washes out in one shampoo.

Semipermanent tints and dyes are highlighters and darkeners; they cannot lighten hair. But they're meant to last through about a month of shampooing before washing out.

The term "permanent hair coloring" includes tinting, lightening, frosting, tipping, streaking, and painting. Permanent coloring means that the color will not wash out but will remain until the hair is cut.

Any pregnant woman who uses permanent hair coloring should be aware of possible allergic reactions that can be caused by chemicals in the product. Because skin may be more sensitive during pregnancy, you may find hair dyes—even the one you've always used before—very irritating. Reactions can include swelling around the eyes, and redness, itching, and burning of facial and neck skin. Permanent dyes produce the largest number of these reactions (though they may not appear until after the dye has been used for some time); semipermanent and temporary colors are generally not irritating.

Semipermanent and permanent dyes contain a statement that a "patch test" should be performed before the hair is colored. This test involves placing a small amount of the dye on an unobtrusive skin area, such as inside the arm, then waiting twenty-four to forty-eight hours to see if any reaction occurs. This test is particularly important if you are pregnant. Since sensitivity to dyes can occur at any time, a patch test done before every coloring can prevent major irritation from a complete dyeing.

Hair dyes and the fetus

In addition to allergic reactions, some pregnant women may be worried about possible effects hair dyes have on the fetus. Their concern is based on testimony by the Environmental Defense Fund before Congress that certain ingredients in hair dyes caused birth defects in lab animals. Other tests, however, seem to show that suspect substances in hair dyes do *not* cause birth defects in test animals. The question is undecided, and some cosmetics companies, such as Clairol, have removed controversial ingredients from their products. Major cosmetics companies we contacted said that using their hair-coloring products poses no risk to the fetus.

Another type of permanent dye that has become more popular recently is henna. This natural vegetable dye rarely produces allergic reactions and is quite safe to use in all other respects.

Besides allergic reactions, damage to hair is a major consideration for pregnant women who permanently color their hair, simply because their hair strands may already be weakened. Permanent dyes and bleaches are generally alkalinic preparations that dry and slightly damage hair with each application. Too frequent or drastic color changes can be harsh on hair, and lead to dullness and split ends. Completely changing your color with a dye or bleach obviously subjects your hair to greater likelihood of damage than frosting or streaking, and has to be done more frequently to maintain a "fresh" look (roots begin to show in about four weeks). One-step coloring products are less harmful than two-step processes. From the standpoint of hair health, pregnant women who experience hair loss or drier-than-usual hair would probably do best to avoid permanent coloring—it can only worsen already weak hair.

Taking care of tinted hair

If you do choose to color or bleach your hair permanently during pregnancy, minimize some of the possible damage by using a mild shampoo—one that's slightly acidic and created for tinted hair is best. Condition after each shampoo. Treat hair periodically to a hot-oil conditioning. At home you can use a product specially created for this conditioning; or heat a small amount of oil, coat your hair, then wrap it in a hot towel for about fifteen minutes; shampoo thoroughly afterward. Use a blow dryer, electric rollers, and curling irons as little as possible. Protect hair from seasonal assaults, such as sun and cold wind (keep hair covered), and chlorinated and salt water (rinse right after swimming).

Keep in mind that if you change your hair tones, your normal makeup may no longer look exactly right. And if pregnancy causes your skin to look sallower, as it sometimes does, a hair color that used to look great may now contrast too much with, or emphasize, the yellow tones in your skin.

Hair waving and straightening

Permanenting and straightening are two other chemical processes that are best avoided during pregnancy if you have weakened hair. Both processes chemically change the molecular structure of the hair. They can make hair dry and brittle if the waving and straightening are done incorrectly or too often.

During pregnancy, chemically curled or straightened hair needs the extra attention you should give to permanently colored hair. Also, even the strongest hair suffers some damage when it is waved, then colored (optimally, one to two weeks later). Hair experts generally feel hair should *never* be straightened, then colored. During pregnancy, decide whether you want your hair curly *or* colored. Waving and straightening are safe during pregnancy, but they can cause allergic reactions. Finally, there is no scientific evidence to support the contention that pregnancy affects the hair's ability to take a permanent wave.

Dry hair

In addition to the problem of hair loss, many women find that their hair is drier during pregnancy, especially during the last trimester. Increased estrogen levels then can cause decreased oil production. Of course, the degree of dryness depends on your prepregnancy hair type—dry, oily, or normal. A woman with typically oily hair may actually find that problem diminished during pregnancy.

If you do experience dry hair, a regimen of gentle care is in order to maintain hair body and manageability, and to prevent dullness and split ends. Wash hair with a shampoo formulated for dry hair. Since even the mildest shampoos are somewhat alkalinic (and thus drying), in order to clean hair, always follow the shampoo with a cream rinse or conditioner (the protein type is best if your hair is thin or damaged). Also, don't overshampoo dry hair. Lather only once and rinse with warm—not hot—water. Some beauty experts suggest adding a little oil to your shampoo to counteract drying agents. An occasional hot-oil treatment and scalp massage may also help relieve some of the dryness.

If at all possible, blow-drying should be avoided if you have dry hair. If you can't avoid it, keep the drying time brief and the temperature low. Curling irons and electric rollers can also wreak havoc; use them infrequently and try a mist setting if possible.

Overbrushing is detrimental to dry hair, too. Two dozen

strokes with a soft-bristle brush each day are more than enough. Brush rollers can be hazardous to dry hair—wearing them too often or too tightly can precipitate some hair loss. Many women no longer use hair spray, either because today's hairstyles often don't require it or because of ecological concern, but chemicals in hair sprays can also cause already dry hair to become even drier. As we've mentioned earlier, chemical processes are best left until after pregnancy if your hair is too dry.

Weather and dry hair

Expectant mothers should give their hair special care during extremes of hot and cold weather. In winter, cover your head well to protect against the temperatures and winds that may rob hair of moisture and make it brittle. Adequate indoor moisture will also benefit dryish hair. In the summer, limit exposure to the sun and wear a hat or scarf to ward off brittleness. Chlorinated and salt water—two other drying agents—should be thoroughly rinsed or shampooed from hair after each swim. In both very hot and very cold weather, redouble conditioning. Protein conditioners and oil treatments will guard against potential weather hazards and are essential to hair's luster and manageability, especially if it's dry or treated chemically.

Finally, easy-to-style hair is always a good idea during pregnancy, when your time as well as your desire and even your ability to fuss with your hair may hit a new low. A simple style—one that doesn't have to be teased, blown, curled, and sprayed all the time—will eliminate much of the manipulation that worsens dry hair. If you're suffering with split ends, an often attendant problem, a no-nonsense cut is essential.

Oily hair

During pregnancy, some women feel their hair is oilier than at other times, though this problem is not as prevalent as that of dry hair. Again, your problem will depend on your original hair type—dry, normal, or oily—but increased levels of progesterone may make hair oilier, and hormonal stimulation of sweat glands during pregnancy may cause hair to feel drab and limp.

If your hair does seem oilier during pregnancy, get an easy-care, shorter hairstyle that can withstand frequent washing. When you shampoo—and do so as often as your hair needs it—use a brand formulated for oily hair, with warm rather than hot water, and lather twice. Try leaving the second application on for a few minutes to remove excess oils thoroughly. Rinsing with cool water or a homemade vinegar or lemon-juice preparation may also cut down on your hair's oiliness. Unless you really need conditioners for manageability and can find one especially made for oily hair, avoid them. Most contain substances such as balsam and protein that when added to natural oil tend to make hair dull and dirty.

With blow-drying, the hottest settings may stimulate oil production, so use a warm or cool setting instead. Beauty experts disagree as to the amount of brushing that oily hair should receive. Some believe overbrushing may increase oil production, while others feel a complete brushing is vital to hair, oily or not. Excessively oily hair may also be helped by brief sunlamp treatments, but these should be done only after consulting a doctor, and the physician's directions should be followed explicitly. The rays emitted from a sunlamp are as safe for pregnant women as they are for nonpregnant women.

Skin

Your skin, like most other organs of your body, undergoes enormous changes during pregnancy—although these changes are highly individual and unpredictable. One of the best known is called *chloasma* (klo-az'-ma), or "mask of pregnancy": melanin or brown pigmentation in skin increases, resulting in dark patches on the cheeks, forehead, arms, and around the nipples. Existing freckles and moles may darken, and new ones may appear. This condition is related to high levels of estrogen and progesterone, and can begin a few weeks after conception and last the entire pregnancy. Brunettes seem to be more subject to this increased pigmentation.

Most specialists agree there's not much that can be done to get rid of chloasma. Commercial bleaching creams may lighten the affected area, if it's not too large. With chloasma, especially if you're using bleaching creams, it's important to stay out of the direct sun (whether in summer or on a bright winter day) to avoid further skin darkening. If you must be in the sun, consult your doctor about a preparation that will block the sun's rays. With today's huge assortment of cosmetic preparations, chloasma can be better endured by using a concealing stick with makeup base over it.

Dry skin

Another pregnancy problem that may affect face and body

skin is dryness. The increased estrogen that dries your hair now can also dry your skin. Too much summer sun, or drying winter wind, or even excessive air conditioning, can aggravate this condition by robbing the skin of much-needed moisture.

For facial skin that may even seem more sensitive than body skin during pregnancy, wash (not too often) with a mild soap—one without deodorant or scent, both of which may be irritating. Many women report that scented soap and even their usual cologne or perfume does not "sit" just right during pregnancy. So you may have to try another brand or stop wearing a particular scent altogether during that time. Cleansing with cold creams may remove some surface dirt without drying, but they do not clean as effectively as soap. Regular use of a nongreasy moisturizing cream (not cold cream) after washing, under makeup, and at night will also curb that dry, tight feeling on your face.

Dry-skin sufferers should also be wary of overusing astringents and skin fresheners, whose alcohol content may increase dryness; a witch-hazel solution is fine. Oil- and cream-based makeup—for the face, lips, and eyes—is best if your skin is dry. The cream in the makeup will help delay moisture loss from skin, and provide smoothness, too. Avoid powder on your face and eyes—it tends to remove moisturizers that are especially needed by dryish skin. You can reintroduce moisture to your dry skin with a face mask that cleans away dirt and dead cells, and helps slow moisture evaporation from skin. Carefully exposing your face to a few minutes of steam treatment—using a towel over a bowl of hot water—will also moisturize skin.

Oily skin

Women with oily skin usually find this condition improves during pregnancy. With decreased oil production, blemishes may also decrease, and these women may discover their complexions are better than ever during the prenatal period. Nevertheless, some women actually feel their facial skin is oilier when they're pregnant. Whether this is the result of higher progesterone levels or increased perspiration during pregnancy, there are steps that can be taken. Start by washing frequently with soap, and rinse with lukewarm or cool water. Whatever soap your skin will tolerate is fine, although your doctor or druggist can recommend a brand designed specifically for oily skin. Follow the washings with an application of astringent for further cleansing and skin toning. If you can't wash with soap during the day as often as your skin needs it, carry a package of cleansing towelettes for convenience.

Be especially careful to clean away all makeup at night. A weekly application of a cleansing pack can provide a thorough scrubbing for oily skin and prevent clogged pores. Commercial scrubs are available, or you can make your own by mixing oatmeal and water into a paste. Apply the pack to your face, then rinse thoroughly with cool water. Creams and oils in any form will only aggravate your problem by helping to seal oil into your skin; use water-based foundation and apply with a moist sponge. Cut down on moisturizers. Powdered products will help remove some of the excess oil from your skin, but in extreme cases of oiliness your doctor may prescribe sunlamp treatments.

Contrary to the notion about pregnancy "glow," some women complain of a sallow or lifeless complexion during that time. Fatigue, stress, and your body's need for more iron can contribute to a "washed-out" look. Extra rest, if possible, and a balanced diet may help, and some experts feel that body toning exercise or yoga may bring color back, at least temporarily, to your cheeks.

Pregnancy makeup tips from cosmetic designer Marilyn Miglin, president of Marilyn Miglin Model Makeup, Inc., Chicago:

1. Apply foundation with a moist sponge, starting with a fingertip's worth in the center of the cheeks and fanning out. Blend lightly.

2. Women with oily skin should use water-based makeup; women with dry skin should use oil-based cosmetics.

3. For the sallow skin of pregnancy, use transparent colored liquid under or in place of base. (The base adds a protective covering for your skin.)

4. If your lips are especially dry, be sure to use lip gloss every day.

5. Skin changes may mean a makeup switch; try out new kinds—*not* on the backs of the hands but on the skin around your collarbone.

6. Pregnancy may be the time for a soft look. Avoid brassy tones and harsh black eyeliner. Try pale, neutral shadows, off-pink-beige tones, and soft brown liners.

7. Because your body is continuously changing, periodically rethink your cosmetic needs.

8. To minimize puffiness around the eyes, use dark-gray or dark-brown shadow along the orbital bone area, then lighten the lid to create an illusion of depth.

9. A rouge darker than your usual shade, applied with a brush under your cheekbones, will minimize the appearance of puffiness.

10. If you have the "mask of pregnancy" and plan to be in the sun, make up as follows: first apply sunscreen (pay careful attention to the high cheek area, the tops of brows, and the mustache area), then add a cream-base makeup.

11. If your nails become more brittle, use a nail conditioner and fortifier.

12. Don't make up for the day until nausea subsides.

Eye care

Your eyes and the delicate skin around them can also be affected by your pregnancy. Sensitive tissues surrounding the eyes may be drier now. Take special care of this area with creamy moisturizers at night and under your makeup during the day. A sunscreen on top of those moisturizers is a good idea, too, if you'll be out in glaring summer or winter sun. When making up or removing makeup from the eyelids or the area beneath the eyes, work gently to prevent further damage to dry, tender skin there. Puffiness may appear around your eyes as part of the normal edema, or accumulation of fluids, in your body during pregnancy. Try placing small pads dipped in cold water on your eyelids or under your eyes to reduce swelling. Some women normally have dark circles or lines under their eyes. During pregnancy, these may seem more prominent, especially if the skin is paler than usual. A good diet and sufficient rest will serve your entire complexion well during pregnancy, and will definitely help to deemphasize the dark circles. If you still find the circles too unsightly, dab them lightly with a *small* amount of cover-stick or liquid makeup base.

Stretch marks

Stretch marks, or *striae* (stry'-ee), are caused by the breaking of tissue under the skin as it stretches to meet the demands of pregnancy, and are also hormonally induced. Fair-skinned women seem to be particularly susceptible. These reddish streaks generally appear on the abdomen, breasts, and thighs and become permanent whitish marks after delivery. Unfortunately, nothing seems to make stretch marks disappear once they occur. But everyone seems to have a different opinion on preventing them. Some experts feel that stretch marks will occur or not depending on the skin's elasticity and ability to endure the rapid weight gain of pregnancy. They believe that no amount of lotion or cream applied to the skin can really prevent damage. Others feel that frequent massage with moisturizing creams or cocoa butter, and watching fat intake and weight gain, can at least reduce the severity of stretch marks.

Breast care

Besides stretch marks, you will probably observe many changes in your breasts during pregnancy. They will most likely enlarge, which may mean you'll need more support than you're used to in a bra. As pregnancy progresses, the veins of your breasts will become more prominent, and nipples and areola—the area around the nipples—often will darken. From mid-pregnancy onward (though some women do not experience it until immediately after the baby's birth), your nipples may secrete a yellowish fluid known as *colostrum* (kuh-lahs'-truhm). Before your milk comes in, this substance provides vitamins, protein, and antibodies beneficial to your baby. The amount of colostrum secreted during pregnancy may be negligible, or it may be enough to warrant wearing breast shields or other absorbent material to protect your clothing. Rinsing with water (no soap) should be sufficient to keep colostrum from becoming sticky on skin and clothing.

Contrary to advice in the past, breasts generally do not need special care during most of your pregnancy. However, if you plan to nurse your baby, it's a good idea in the last couple of months to prepare your nipples somewhat for the "exercise" they will receive from your newborn. Avoid washing your nipples and areola with soap or other strong cleaning solutions such as alcohol. Rinsing only with water will not rob nipples of natural moisture secretions. There seems to be no foolproof method of toughening nipples during pregnancy to prevent discomfort during nursing. Advice on using a brush or rubbing with a rough cloth has been discredited, though some women feel that periodically exposing their nipples to the air after washing reduces tenderness later. Applying moisturizing creams and lotions to nipples has no proved value for later nursing comfort.

Your body

Like your facial skin, your body skin may be more sensitive and dry during pregnancy. Some women even experience a general itchiness all over their bodies. To counteract dryness, wash with a mild, unscented, unmedicated soap, and don't overclean. For example, shower rather than bathe, or make your baths briefer. Try to avoid very hot water.

Bath oils, used occasionally, may also help with dry skin, though some experts feel the perfume may be irritating to sensitive genital skin and cause symptoms simulating urinary tract infections. Be careful with a slippery tub, though, when using bath oils. Bath salts and bubble-bath preparations should be avoided, as they can cause dryness and irritation to sensitive body areas. Bath powders may cause a bit more dryness than you want now.

Removing body hair

Removal of hair from legs and thighs can also irritate dry skin if done too frequently. Many women use a safety razor in the bath, and lather with soap and water, though shaving after the bath with a cream or lotion for lubrication may be better. In either case, and also after using an electric shaver, apply moisturizer generously to the shaved areas. Chemical depilatories (cream, foam, or liquid) are safe for pregnant women. These products do contain strong substances, though, and must be used carefully to avoid skin dryness and irritation. Removing body hair with heated wax is also safe, but probably should be done by a professional. Electrolysis should also be performed by an expert. Though it is safe, electrolysis can be a time-consuming and somewhat uncomfortable procedure, one that most women would probably want to forgo during pregnancy.

Sunbathing

Like your hair, your dry skin deserves special consideration during weather that can make it even drier. If you want to sunbathe, do so only for brief periods, always using a sunscreen preparation (even on cloudy days) that will protect your skin. The most effective sunscreens contain para-amino benzoic acid (PABA) or a salicylate. If you burn very easily (and many women are more prone to sunburn during pregnancy), have your doctor prescribe a preparation that will almost totally block the sun's rays. After sunning, dry skin requires generous moisturizing with a cream or lotion.

If you want color without sun, in summer or winter, it's safe to apply artificial tanning products that are not systemically absorbed. Just be aware that they may cause an allergic reaction and that prolonged use may promote more dryness.

Cold weather

Extremely cold weather can cause as much damage to dry skin as the hot summer sun. Make sure your skin is well protected and don't squeeze moisture from your dry skin by soaking in a hot tub. Again, try to shower, or make your baths short. Moisturizing is a must now—use a nongreasy cream or lotion all over your body after every bath, after shaving, after you've been outdoors for a prolonged period, and before bed. You can also aid dry skin by making sure your indoor environment contains plenty of humidity.

Perspiration

Many women perspire more during pregnancy. Even if your skin is generally drier now, you can at least use a deodorant soap on your underarms.

Saunas

Many persons enjoy sauna baths. But pregnant women should avoid them. Not only are they generally drying to skin, but recent studies done by researchers at the University of Washington School of Medicine in Seattle suggest that saunas in early pregnancy may produce brain damage in the fetus.

Vaginal care

During pregnancy, vaginal secretions can increase, and often make you feel uncomfortable. If your discharge is caused by an infection, your doctor can prescribe a particular treatment (see page 61).

For the normal vaginal moisture that sometimes accompanies pregnancy, regular washing of the vulvar area with water and mild, unscented, nondeodorant soap will help you stay fresh and minimize an odor problem. Wear absorbent cotton or cotton-panel panties to help reduce stickiness during the day. A variety of small sanitary pads now on the market will also soak up discharge in a relatively unobtrusive fashion. (Tampons are not a good idea; the congestion of the vagina may make them uncomfortable.) At night, try to sleep without panties.

Vaginal deodorant sprays, which were in vogue several years ago, have been shown to be potentially harmful to delicate vaginal tissues. Douching to cure vaginal discharge has also been discredited and may destroy beneficial bacteria that are needed to fight harmful organisms in the vagina. Douching may even increase the amount of discharge. Pregnant women should never use a bulb syringe to douche because of the danger of air embolism.

CHAPTER THIRTEEN
Dressing the Part:
The Maternity Wardrobe

It may not happen in the third month, or even in the fourth, but one day early in your pregnancy it will. You unfold a favorite pair of jeans and pull them on. You struggle with the zipper and snap before you realize—it's time for maternity clothes.

When?

Some women want to get into maternity wear early. For them it might be a physical affirmation of pregnancy or a mark of womanliness. They may start wearing maternity clothes as soon as the second month of pregnancy, although at this point, in most cases, the uterus feels like nothing more than a small bump just above the pelvic bone. But maternity clothes are not made to fit the *slightly* pregnant body. Slacks tend to be longer without the poundage that lifts them up. Tops may look baggy because maternity shirts are cut for the usually larger bustline of later pregnancy.

"Clothes tolerance" is another factor to consider before you begin wearing maternity clothing. Maternity wardrobes are generally small, so if you tire of clothes easily, hold off a little on maternity apparel. Outfits you wear for four months seem a lot more attractive than those you've been wearing once a week for seven months. Once you've started maternity wear, don't save the good items for "later." Pregnancy is short enough, and you'll probably feel better with more variety in your wardrobe.

Some women delay getting into maternity clothes until the last possible moment—when they can't wear even the loosest-fitting article in the closet. It's better—both physically and psychologically—to move into maternity wear before it's impossible to wear everyday clothes. Women carrying their first child often go into maternity clothes later than those who have previously delivered. This is because the recti muscles of a woman in her first pregnancy are tight and better able to hold in the expanding uterus. Water weight also influences how comfortable a woman feels.

Each pregnant woman should decide for herself when to start wearing maternity clothes—and not be swayed by the examples of others. Comfort is the key, and most women find they're comfortable in maternity wear somewhere between the third and fifth month.

Maternity styles

It's only fairly recently that maternity clothes have been fashionable. Sacklike smocks, skirts with large, chilly slits (instead of stretch panels), and dresses that looked like tents were the options our mothers had. Maternity specialty shops were rare, and department stores offered a relatively small selection of maternity wear. Women often made do with loose-fitting housecoats at home and larger-sized regular clothes when they went out.

In the late sixties, though, maternity manufacturers got smart, as the postwar baby-boom generation began having their own children. Bright colors, better styling, and decent fabrics started to appear—and soon maternity boutiques sprang up. In a world that is increasingly fashion-conscious, more women are now working outside the home, being active the whole nine months of what women used to think of as a temporary retirement. They want and need much more than formless dresses that could better serve as parachutes. Expectant mothers are often in their mid- to late twenties or thirties and prefer sophisticated clothes to the junior styles of the sixties and before. And they've been finding them in such specialty shops as Lady Madonna, Motherhood Maternity, Mothercare, Maternity Modes, and Page Boy. Today, maternity wear is an $800-million-a-year business.

Just about anything you'd regularly wear comes in a maternity style. Besides a huge variety of maternity mainstays such as tops, slacks, and everyday dresses, the selection includes pants outfits, jeans, jumpers, sweaters, long and short skirts and matching blouses, body suits, full-length evening gowns, swimsuits, tennis and running outfits, shorts, halter tops, sundresses, beach cover-ups, coats, slickers, capes, ponchos, bras, slips, hose, girdles, nightgowns, and robes. Maternity clothes are available in fabrics to fit most preferences and all seasons. Of course, it isn't always necessary to get clothing geared specifically for pregnancy. Whatever clothing you feel good in should be what you wear during pregnancy.

Tops

Maternity tops are available in five styles: A-line, Empire, pleated, smock, and tie-in-the-back, with a variety of sleeve lengths. Depending on your weight gain, build, and how you carry the baby, you may feel more comfortable in a particular blouse style. Most women buy or acquire more tops than pants for a pregnancy, since what covers your abdomen seems to be the focal point of what you wear. Make sure blouses (and dress tops) fit well around the neck and shoulders. A good fit in those areas can make you feel neater and less as though the top is engulfing you (a common clothes complaint, especially in early pregnancy).

Sweaters

There's a wide choice in maternity sweaters now, too: bulky knit and thin-ribbed, cowl and turtleneck, for example. Because of nausea or shortness of breath, many women find sweaters that fit loosely around the neck more comfortable. It's probably best not to buy maternity sweaters in anticipation of cold weather. Many women, even those who are normally "cold-blooded," find themselves much warmer as they gain weight and undergo other physical changes. Wait to see how you feel; then choose your sweater weights accordingly. Some regular sweater styles will adapt well to your maternity needs: cardigans left unbuttoned, long pullovers, turtlenecks worn under jumpers or maternity tops.

Dresses

As we've noted, almost every imaginable dress style is available in maternity wear, whether you need something for a formal wedding or a casual summer picnic. Many women prefer dresses during their pregnancies, especially if they work outside the home, if the weather is warm (and they're feeling even warmer), or if their weight gain makes slacks seem binding. Some women also report that dresses make them feel more attractive than slacks do.

Pants

Most maternity slacks accommodate your growing abdomen with a front panel of stretchy fabric. This panel can appear in pants of any fabric—wool, cotton, polyester. An alternative is maternity slacks made completely of a stretchy material—with more fabric in front—so that the entire garment expands as you do. This type might be more comfortable for certain body contours. Some women, however, find the material never expands as much as does the stretch panel in traditional maternity slacks. Others say that if the fabric is too conforming to the figure, every lump and bump in the thighs shows through. Whatever the construction, slacks may be more comfortable during cold weather or more appealing if your legs are particularly swollen or you have prominent varicose veins.

Jumpers

Jumpers are versatile. Depending on color and fabric, many jumpers can be worn sleeveless during warm weather, with a light blouse when it's cooler, and with a sweater or body suit on the coldest days.

Specialty items

The appearance of such specialty items as maternity swimsuits, tennis dresses, and running suits reflects the revolution in maternity clothes. Take advantage. If swimming and tennis are normally part of your life, it's important to get the clothes you need to feel comfortable continuing these activities during your pregnancy.

Bras

Basically, there are two types of bra you might buy when you're pregnant. Some manufacturers offer *maternity* bras. Some are no different from the nonmaternity type, so you might as well wear what you're accustomed to. Other maternity bras are made to "give" during pregnancy. If they do, they may not provide proper support. Maternity bras are all nylon or a cotton blend, with varying degrees of decoration. Like most maternity foundation garments, maternity bras are white, with beige occasionally available.

Nursing bras feature fasteners on the straps that allow the cups, or a panel on the cups, to unhook for easy breast-feeding. Some women complain, though, that the flap arrangement on some nursing bras is bulky and unattractive under clothes. Nursing bras are all cotton or all nylon; some have underwires for extra support. To ensure a comfortable fit, it's probably best not to buy nursing bras until close to delivery.

Whether to wear a bra at all, or whether to change bra types during pregnancy and lactation, are topics that warrant some consideration. If your breasts do not change drastically while you're pregnant and nursing, there's no medical reason to start wearing a bra then if you haven't before. Some women report, though, that they did feel better, at least during the first weeks of nursing, with some support. In this case, two bras packed for the hospital might be all you need. Your regular bras may fit well during pregnancy. In a few cases, regular bras may fit well even during nursing, and are especially convenient if they're the front-hooking type. Some women also use their regular back-hooking bras during nursing, and just pull up the entire cup when the baby must be fed.

Comfort is crucial, whether or not you wear a bra during pregnancy and lactation. You can probably go through early pregnancy with your regular-size bra. Many women then increase one cup size and one back size during the rest of pregnancy. If you buy a bra during pregnancy, have it fitted carefully: make sure the straps don't dig in, the back doesn't ride up as you move, the cups don't cut under your breasts. Also see that the front panels of nursing bras unfasten with ease. Bra sizes generally range from 32A to 42F, though some large department stores can have even larger sizes specially made.

Panties

Maternity underpants either are made from a stretchy material or are all cotton, nylon tricot, or acetate tricot panties with stretch front panels. They are available in a full brief style (no bikinis) in "one size fits all" or sizes small to extra large. White is the most common color, although you may be able to find some pastels. Always buy panties with a cotton crotch—they allow air flow to the genital area, which is especially important during pregnancy. Maternity panties are not a *necessity*, though. Many women get through pregnancy with regular briefs or bikinis, depending on their comfort and stretchability.

Girdles

Maternity girdles come in pantie, regular-support, and back-support styles, and they are fitted according to hip size (measuring under the baby). In the past, many doctors recommended a girdle as a regular part of prenatal care, to maintain muscle tone or relieve backache during pregnancy. Today, however, most pregnant women forgo girdles of any kind, feeling they are constrictive and uncomfortable. Unless you always wear a girdle or your physician prescribes one for a specific problem, you needn't be outfitted for a maternity girdle.

Slips

Depending on cut and fabric, many regular slips will fit during pregnancy. If you don't want to run the risk of stretching out your everyday slips, though, half-slips, full slips, and even formal-length slips are available in maternity styles. Most prenatal slips come in white nylon tricot with front stretch panels, and are measured according to bra size for a full slip, and hip size for a half-slip.

Hosiery

Some women claim that queen-size panty hose (for larger, not taller, figures) fits well during pregnancy. (Queen-size panty hose is also cheaper than the maternity variety.) Maternity hose is sized according to height and weight, and comes in a variety of shades. Sheer maternity hose is less expensive than support maternity hose, which offers support in the legs, or in the legs *and* in a front panel. If your legs are especially achy during pregnancy, support hose may relieve the problem; if your uterine ligaments ache, support hose with a support front panel may help.

Nightwear

There is a variety of attractive styles, fabrics, and colors available in maternity nightwear. Most of us, though, don't buy new gowns and robes just for pregnancy unless our regular ones become too tight. In that case, you can choose between a maternity style and a looser-fitting, regular one. If you plan to nurse your baby, you need gowns, pajamas, and robes that open easily. Many women choose regular nightwear that unbuttons, unzips, or "flips" open for easy nursing. Special nursing gowns are also made with a hidden opening for breast-feeding. Because nursing gowns are cut very full, consider purchasing and wearing nursing nightwear during pregnancy. If you choose maternity styles, make sure they will be adaptable to nursing later on, if you plan to breast-feed.

Shoes

Finally, a word about shoes, although they're not specifically fashioned for maternity use. For most women, comfort in shoes seems especially important during pregnancy. Lower heels, wider toes, and nonskid soles make sense at this time, when you might be more prone to fatigue, leg aches, swollen feet, and varicose veins. Toward the end of pregnancy, slip-on shoes may be ideal, because bending over to tie laces or clasp buckles becomes increasingly difficult.

Cost of maternity clothes

The styles, colors, and fabrics of maternity clothes have improved over the years. But even though you'll wear maternity clothes for less than nine months, you probably won't be paying any less for their lack of longevity. For example, attractive maternity tops range in price from $15 to $45; pants, from $20 to $60; and dresses, from $25 to $100. In expensive maternity shops, however, you may pay even more. Maternity clothes are sometimes less sturdy than the same articles in regular styles. Manufacturers assume women won't be wearing them long enough for them to fall apart.

Obvious alternatives to buying a completely new wardrobe include borrowing from friends and scouring recycled clothes shops (for more information, see page 209). Unfortunately, maternity shop sales are infrequent, and the odds are against finding price reductions on what you want when you need it. If you're expecting your first baby and you know you'll have more, or if you're on your third or fourth and feel it's time for a new set of clothes, then a new wardrobe makes sense.

Planning before you purchase is a good principle to follow with a maternity wardrobe. Before you shop, take a thorough survey of what you already have. What will see you comfortably through the first few months? What can you adapt for maternity wear later?

When you do begin shopping, your own taste will take over. You know what you like and what looks best on you. These days, you might even be able to completely outfit yourself happily in maternity fashions. But bear in mind a few tips:

• Make each piece of maternity apparel as versatile as possible.
• Select colors within the same family.
• Choose clothes that "layer." They'll make the best wardrobe expanders.

• Don't buy clothes with the intention of wearing them after the baby is born.

Chic, all-season maternity wardrobes

To help in planning your purchases to maximize your dollars, we offer six sample wardrobes for "pregnancy seasons." The average wardrobe listed costs around $400, a figure that does not include a winter coat (for those who need one), underwear, or accessories. (See page 208 for an underwear guide.) Costs vary, of course, according to fabrics, the stores you shop in, and how many items you buy that we recommend (some seasons call for more clothes than others, depending on how easily you can layer). You may not wish to spend this sum, and so will trim the list, or you may wish to spend much more. The point is, the list has the basics, which you can adapt to meet your own needs.

The wardrobes are meant both for women who work outside the home and those who work in the home (although more dresses are recommended for women who have jobs outside the home). Today, there's not a radical difference in the clothing demands of the two life-styles. Those who care for children and a home are as active as women who hold jobs for pay. So, nearly every expectant mother needs a multipurpose wardrobe.

Finally, when using the sample wardrobes, remember that "seasons" means the seasons of the north and middle sectors of the United States, where winters are cold, falls crisp, springs cool, and summers hot. Of course, a pregnancy spans several seasons; each of the sample wardrobes takes weather changes into account through the number, type, and fabric of the garments. Also, the kinds of clothes and fabrics mentioned are based on the assumption that you'll start wearing maternity clothes around the beginning of the fourth month of pregnancy. Make an individual adjustment if you go into maternity apparel earlier or later.

• *Winter*
Your due date: December–January
You start wearing maternity clothes: June–July

Nonmaternity clothes to wear in the early months:

beltless dresses
tunic tops
loose jumpers
peasant blouses

slit-sided shirts
Oshkosh overalls
shirts with drawstring bottoms
slacks with drawstring or elastic waists
wraparound skirts

Maternity clothes you'll need:

3 pairs cotton, light synthetic, or light cotton-blend slacks
2 pairs corduroy, denim, heavy synthetic, or heavy cotton-blend slacks
1 pair wool or wool-blend slacks
3 cotton, light synthetic, or light cotton-blend tops
3 heavy synthetic or heavy cotton-blend tops
1 denim slacks outfit
1 corduroy or denim jumper
1 cotton, light synthetic, or light cotton-blend dress
1 heavy synthetic or heavy cotton-blend dress*

You'll be facing cold weather for at least two months; it's probably worth purchasing a loose-fitting or maternity winter coat.

• *Winter–Spring*
Your due date: February–March
You start wearing maternity clothes: August–September

Nonmaternity clothes to wear in the early months:

loose-fitting sundresses
summer smock dresses
linen drawstring slacks
beach cover-ups
maillots
two-piece bathing suits
terry-cloth shirts
tennis dress rather than shorts
running shorts

---

* For each listed wardrobe, the working woman should purchase several additional dresses if her job demands them.

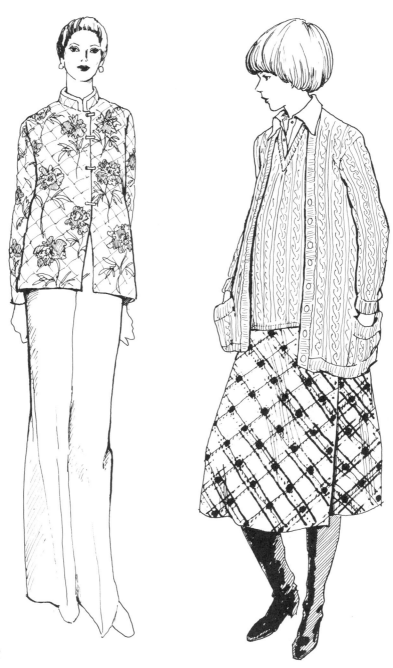

Winter

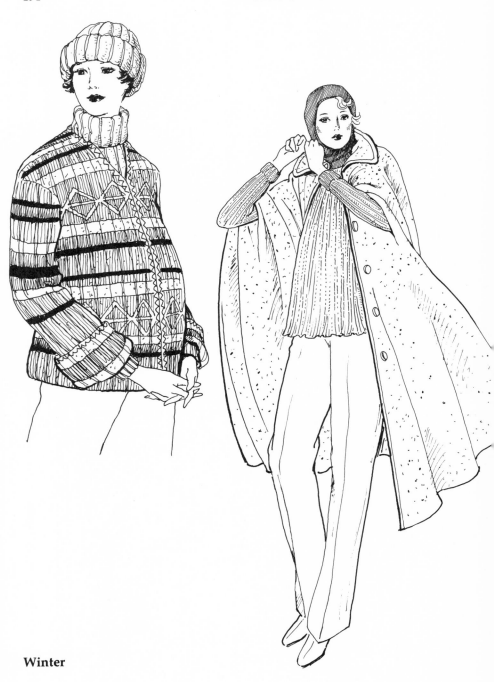

Winter

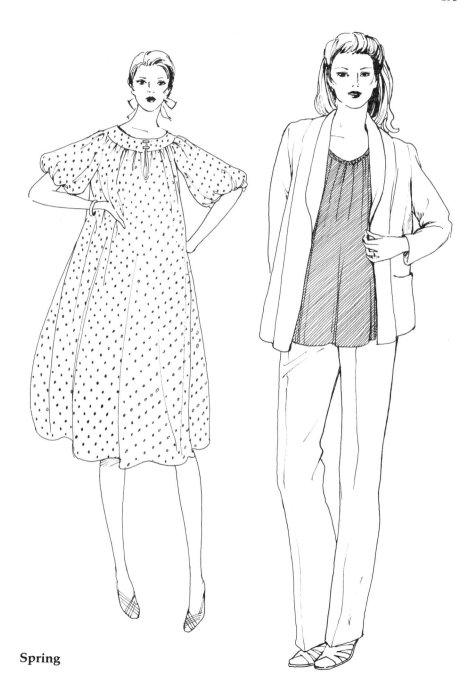

Spring

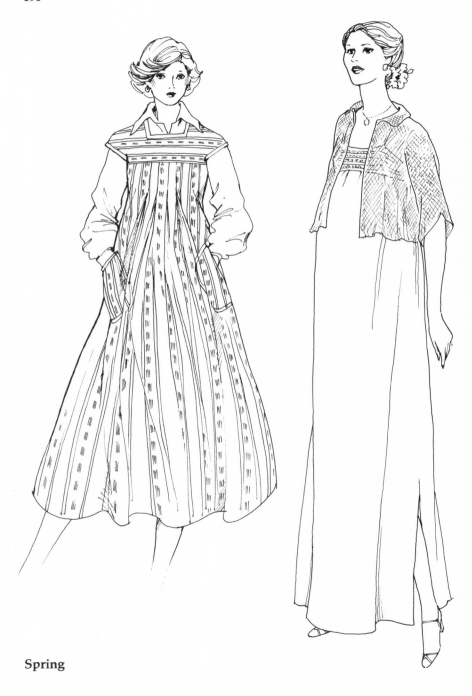

Spring

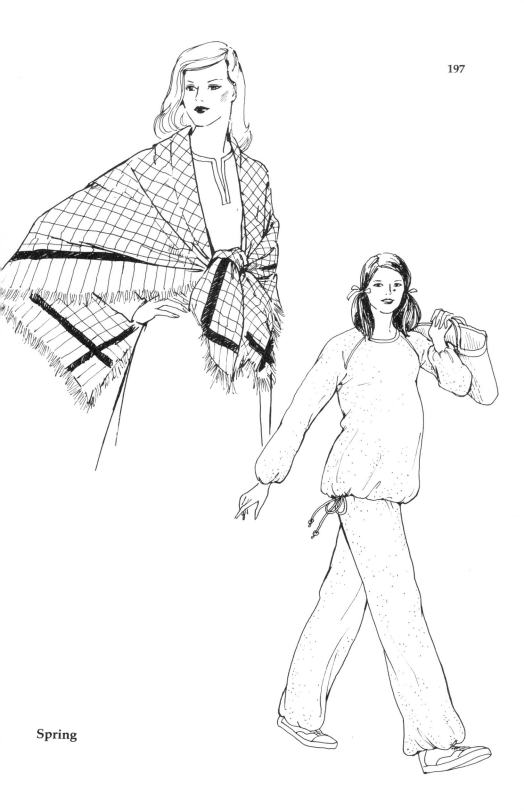

Spring

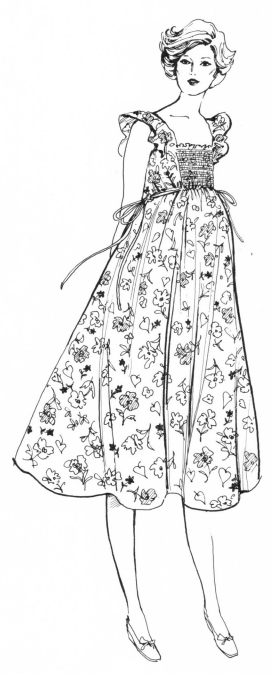

Summer

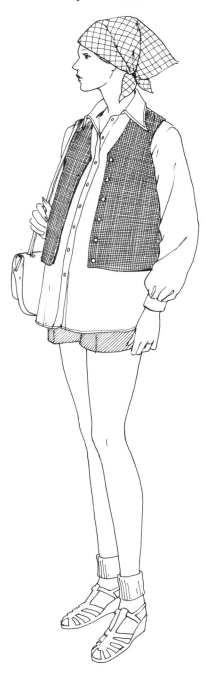

Summer

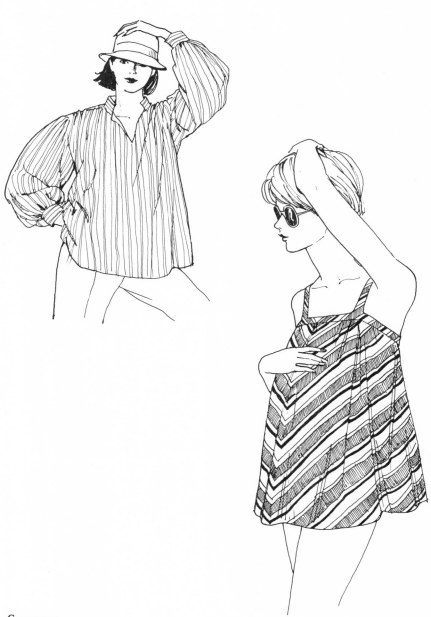

Summer

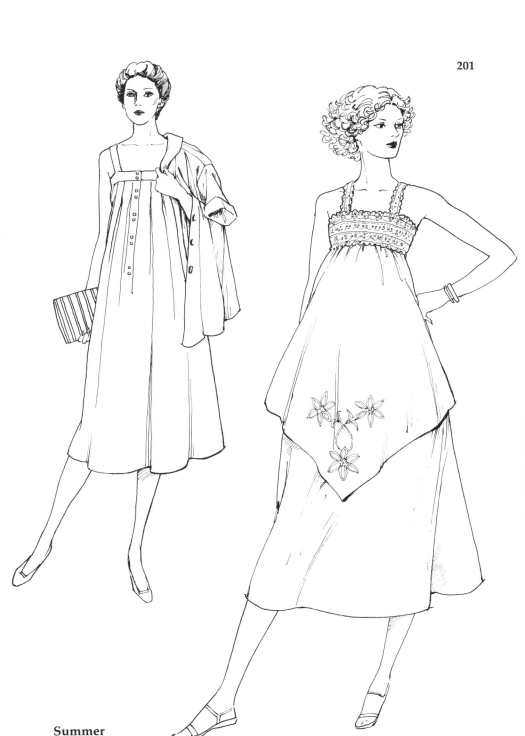

Summer

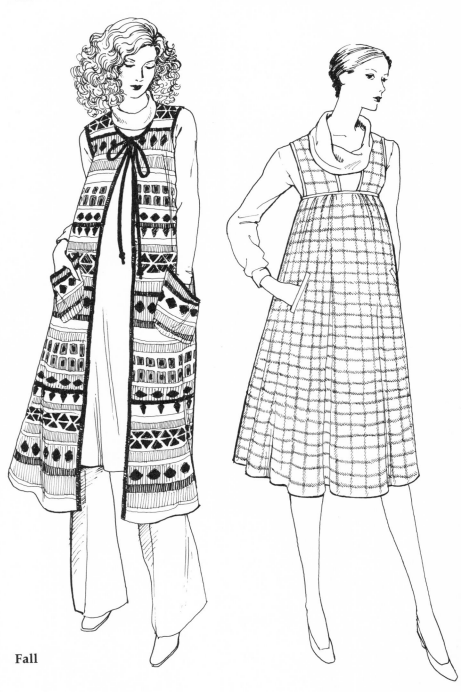

Fall

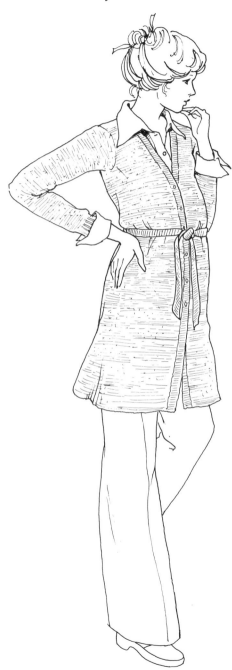

Fall

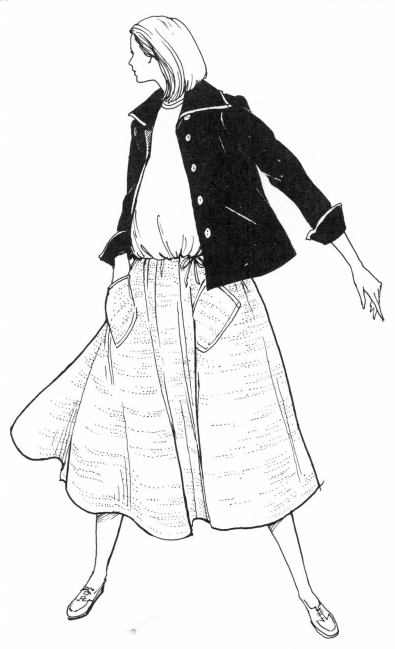

Fall

Maternity clothes you'll need:

1 pair cotton or light cotton-blend slacks
3 pairs corduroy, denim, or heavy synthetic or heavy cotton-blend slacks
1 pair wool or wool-blend slacks
2 cotton, light synthetic, or light cotton-blend layerable tops
3 heavy synthetic or heavy cotton-blend tops
1 corduroy or denim slacks outfit
1 corduroy or denim jumper
1 heavy synthetic, heavy cotton-blend, wool or wool-blend dress

February–March will be your due date; most women will find they will need an especially large winter coat if December, January, and February are cold months.

•Spring

Your due date: April–May
You start wearing maternity clothes: October–November

Nonmaternity clothes to wear in the early months:

Indian or gauzelike shirts
elastic-waisted cotton slacks
sundresses
shirred cotton skirts
windbreakers
velour running suits
corduroy and denim jumpers
shawls
cardigans

Maternity clothes you'll need:

3 pairs corduroy, denim, heavy synthetic, or heavy cotton-blend slacks
1 pair cotton or light cotton-blend slacks
3 heavy synthetic or heavy cotton-blend tops to layer
2 cotton, light synthetic, or light cotton-blend layerable tops

1 cotton slacks outfit
1 wool or wool-blend slacks outfit
1 denim or corduroy jumper
1 wool or wool-blend dress

Some women may need a large coat to see them through the winter. Don't buy one until you are well into your pregnancy. It's difficult to gauge now how much weight you will gain until at least the sixth or seventh month, and you might make a costly mistake.

• Summer

Your due date: June–July
You start wearing maternity clothes: December–January

Nonmaternity clothes to wear in the early months:

corduroy jumpers
cardigans
knit slacks
beltless dresses
shawls
Mexican bulky knit sweaters
Fisherman knit sweaters

Maternity clothes you'll need:

2 pairs wool or wool-blend slacks
2 pairs cotton, light synthetic, or light cotton-blend slacks
1 pair corduroy slacks
2 cotton, light synthetic, or light cotton-blend layerable tops
3 flannel or wool or wool-blend tops
1 corduroy slacks outfit
1 corduroy or denim jumper
1 wool or wool-blend dress
1 cotton, light synthetic, or light cotton-blend dress

You won't be delivering until June or July, so you won't be at your largest until the winter has passed. You will not, then, ordinarily need to purchase a maternity winter coat, although if the spring is cool, you might need a large raincoat. If you can borrow an unshaped raincoat, or move buttons on your own, you'll be prepared.

• Summer–Fall
Your due date: August–September
You start wearing maternity clothes: February–March

Nonmaternity clothes to wear in the early months:

> hooded stretch pullovers
> bulky sweaters
> wool kilts
> stretchable knit slacks
> wool dirndl skirts
> wool jumpers

Maternity clothes you'll need:

> 2 pairs denim, corduroy, heavy synthetic, or heavy cotton-blend slacks
> 3 pairs cotton, light synthetic, or light cotton-blend slacks
> 3 heavy cotton tops
> 3 cotton, light synthetic, or light cotton-blend layerable tops
> 1 corduroy slacks outfit
> 1 corduroy or denim jumper
> 1 cotton, light synthetic, or light cotton-blend dress
> 1 heavy synthetic or heavy cotton-blend dress

Summer–fall mothers can wear regular winter coats and probably never even have to move buttons. If late spring is cool, however, and your raincoat is fitted, you might need a cape or shawl for the chill.

• Fall–Winter
Your due date: October–November
You start wearing maternity clothes: April–May

Nonmaternity clothes to wear in the early months:

cotton dirndl skirts
Mexican bulky knit sweaters for outerwear
shirt jackets
corduroy jumpers
denim jumpers
warm-up clothes

Maternity clothes you'll need:

2 pairs corduroy, denim, heavy synthetic, or heavy cotton-blend slacks
2 pairs cotton, light synthetic, or light cotton-blend slacks
2 heavy cotton, heavy synthetic, or heavy cotton-blend tops
4 cotton, light synthetic, or light cotton-blend tops
1 cotton, light synthetic, or light cotton-blend slacks outfit
1 cotton, light synthetic, or light cotton-blend sundress
1 heavy synthetic or heavy cotton-blend dress
1 denim jumper

If you're giving birth around October, you might find the weather chilly, and you won't be able to fit into your coats. Instead, think about layering, and about using capes and shawls. We advise against purchasing a special winter coat just for November.

• *All seasons underwear and accessories guide*

8 panties (maternity or regular)
6 bras (nursing or regular)
1 slip (maternity or regular)
3 pairs maternity support panty hose
1 maternity bathing suit, if needed
1 maternity tennis dress, if needed
1 maternity warm-up suit, if needed
4 nightgowns (nightgowns adaptable for nursing if you're planning to breast-feed; regular, loose nightgowns if you're not)

Borrowing maternity clothes

Borrowing clothes from friends makes special sense during your pregnancy. Pregnancy is, all in all, a fairly brief period of time. Most women, even those whose clothing budget is unlimited, prefer not to spend enormous sums on clothes they might wear for nine months at most. Depending on specific wardrobe needs, some pregnant women buy several really good items—for work or dressier occasions—and try to fill in with hand-me-downs.

Unlike clothes that are fitted more closely to the body, many maternity pieces can be worn by women of different sizes and shapes. A size 12 woman, for example, may find that her friend's size 9 maternity top fits fine for the early part of her pregnancy. Borrowing may also reduce the boredom you can experience from wearing the same things over and over. Some groups of women even pool their maternity clothes during and after their pregnancies to offer each other a wide selection as the need arises.

Secondhand shops

If you don't have people to borrow from (or don't wish to be a borrower), you still have alternatives to retail buying. Secondhand maternity clothes shops can often be found, especially in larger cities, which usually offer a good selection of recycled items at reduced prices. Many of these stores stock used children's clothing and equipment that can provide additional savings. And it may work the other way around: secondhand children's clothing stores may also carry used maternity clothes.

You may also locate good used maternity wear at church, school, and community rummage sales if you can take the time for sorting through the merchandise. Smaller-scale sales may not offer many items, but other sales are known for their fine selection of maternity clothes and consistently attract large numbers of pregnant women. It's even possible to find maternity wear through house sales, but this is likely to be a much more time-consuming and frustrating search.

Secondhand shops are usually listed in the Yellow Pages or advertised in newspapers. For information on rummage sales, check your local papers and ask knowledgeable friends who've taken advantage of them.

Sewing maternity clothes

Women who can sew are often happier making, rather than buying, their maternity clothes. Despite the wide variety of maternity fashions, sewing your own ensures the fabrics, colors, styles, and fit you want and need. Pattern companies offer a range of patterns for prenatal apparel (see below). Many women with sewing skills design their own maternity clothes or convert some of their regular clothes for maternity wear. If you think you might like to try converting, survey your sewing friends who've been or are pregnant.

Vogue

Six maternity patterns in sizes 8 to 16, including sportswear separates and dresses; some designs by Geoffrey Beene and Lady Madonna; available in department, chain, and specialty stores; no mail order; pattern cost: $2.50 to $4.50.

Butterick

Ten maternity patterns in sizes 8 to 16, including sportswear and separates; available in department, chain, and specialty stores; "See-N-Sew" line also available in some supermarkets and discount stores; pattern cost: $1.25 to $1.75. (Both Butterick and Vogue claim their patterns feature detail work at neck and shoulders, which draws attention to the face and away from the abdomen.)

Simplicity

Ten maternity patterns in sizes 6 to 20, including tops, pants, dresses, jumpers, shorts; available in retail stores; pattern cost: $1.25 to $2.

McCall

Maternity patterns in sizes 8 to 20, including tops, dresses, pants, and shorts; available in department stores, fabric stores, discount stores; pattern cost: $1.25 to $2.

Even amateur sewers can easily change a favorite pair of slacks or shorts (and skirts, too) to maternity styles by cutting out material in the front and inserting a panel of stretchy fabric. Several companies manufacture stretch panels—in a variety of colors—specifically for maternity conversion. Simple directions accompany these panels, which are available in department and fabric stores. If you cannot find the panels in a store near you, try contacting one of the following manufacturers:

E-Z Buckle, Inc.
545 North Arlington Avenue
East Orange, NJ 07017

Belding Lily Company
P.O. Box 88
Shelby, NC 28150

Scovill/Dritz
Buckingham Street
Watertown, CT 06795

Donahue Sales
41 East 31st Street
New York, NY 10022

Mail order

If you have trouble finding maternity clothes where you live, you can mail-order them from some large chain stores. A few of the companies that will mail prepaid maternity clothes across the United States are:

Mothercare-by-Mail
P.O. Box 228
Parsippany, NJ 07054

Maternity tops, pants, dresses, swimsuits, lingerie, and nightwear available through fall–winter and spring–summer catalogs; catalogs can be ordered by mail or found in Mothercare and Mother-To-Be stores across the United States.

Sears, Roebuck and Company
925 South Homan Avenue
Chicago, IL 60607

Write to the address above for the location of your nearest Sears store or Sears catalog order plant; maternity tops, slacks, dresses, swimwear, and some lingerie available through fall–winter and spring–summer catalogs.

J. C. Penney Company, Inc.
11800 West Burleigh Street
Milwaukee, WI 53263

Send $2 for catalog and you will receive with it a $2 gift certificate; maternity tops, pants, dresses, bras, and girdles available through fall–winter and spring–summer catalogs.

Spiegel, Inc.
1061 West 35th Street
Chicago, IL 60609

Send $2 for catalog and you will receive with it a $2 merchandise certificate good for first order; maternity tops, pants, dresses (no lingerie) available through fall–winter and spring–summer catalogs.

Montgomery Ward and Company
Catalog Sales
618 West Chicago Avenue
Chicago, IL 60607

Mail $2 for catalog and receive with it a $2 credit on order; catalog also available through nearest Ward's store; maternity slacks, blouses, dresses, underwear, and hose available through fall–winter and spring–summer catalogs.

Saks Fifth Avenue
611 Fifth Avenue
New York, NY 10022

Special maternity catalog available in January and July at no cost; features tops, pants, dresses, jumpers, skirts, shorts, swimsuits, and nightgowns.

CHAPTER FOURTEEN
On the Job

Working outside the home during pregnancy can be rewarding, an economic necessity, or a way to keep busy. No matter how long you've worked before your pregnancy, your job may be so central to your life that the idea of quitting or cutting back is disturbing. But if you are among the approximately one and a half million women who will work outside the home during pregnancy this year, certainly your pregnancy will affect your job, and in many cases your job may affect your baby.

Physical comfort can be a persistent problem. Women who work at home have access to bathroom, bed, and refrigerator, while access to a lounge on the job may be difficult. Even if the work isn't physically demanding, sitting or standing all day can be more uncomfortable during pregnancy. The overwhelming fatigue that engulfs some women during the first trimester can make a job outside the home uncomfortable or even hazardous, especially if they must drive or operate machinery.

Decisions must be made. How and when to tell your employer that you are pregnant can be a difficult problem. For nine months, many women struggle with the question (self-imposed or otherwise): "Are you coming back after the baby is born?" It seems unfair to have to answer this question just when you must cope with so many other changes in your life.

Besides physical and emotional adjustments, women should consider possible hazards to their babies. Health organizations are beginning to be concerned about on-the-job dangers—chemicals or working conditions—that can harm a fetus or its mother. The pregnant worker today has a special responsibility to be aware of what she breathes, touches, or ingests.

Conflicting emotions: the first trimester

After you discover you are pregnant, joy may commingle with anxiety when you think about your job. As you wonder about the baby, you are bound to consider its effect on your work. While meshing the concepts of "career" and "family" is often difficult, it is particularly so when "family" is nothing more than a positive pregnancy test.

Your sense of proportion may change temporarily. Try as you may to concentrate on your work, you may feel detached from job concerns and spend a lot of time thinking about your unborn child. Many expectant mothers feel guilty for not fully focusing on work.

Although it may be difficult, try not to pressure yourself early in pregnancy about making major decisions, such as how long you will work or whether you will return to the job after the baby's birth. You have many months ahead and a long time to think, read, and talk about these questions with other mothers. Many women have found that problems that seemed perplexing early in pregnancy solved themselves later. If you accept that you'll have ambivalent feelings, you'll find it easier to cope with fleeting insecurities about work and motherhood.

The difficulties aren't only emotional during the first trimester. Women who feel sluggish much of the time can feel ambivalent about work, the baby, or both. If their efficiency has been impaired, they may try to work harder to compensate, or feel guilty or depressed, not realizing that discomforts usually disappear by the fourth month. Nausea takes a toll, too. You feel less than refreshed, and sometimes you look pale and wan. Nausea can diminish concentration and sociability. Again, it's very important to take what steps you can to alleviate the condition and then remember that nausea usually fades by the fourth month.

If your hair and skin are dull, your clothes too tight, and you feel tired, you don't much want to deal with the public. You need to experiment a bit, altering grooming routines until you feel confident again. Getting into attractive maternity clothes can make a difference, too, not only for comfort's sake but because affirming your pregnancy to co-workers and others can boost your spirits and relieve tensions you may have been feeling about "showing."

Some women are irrepressible when they are pregnant. They feel terrific, look terrific, and are elated much of the time. Even if they don't *really* glow, they think they do. This energy spills over into the job. They may feel more creative or think no problem is insurmountable. If they know they will be leaving work eventually, and feel there's not so much at stake as before, they may be more comfortable with superiors or co-workers. This, in turn, may actually improve their job situation.

Of course, it is unlikely that you will sustain a consistent mood or outlook during these nine months, or that your feelings about work will remain constant. You have begun a major transition in your life (particularly if you are expecting your first child). And, like any period of change, this one will be accompanied by shifts and dislocations essential in helping you find a new equilibrium.

Breaking the news

One of the chief considerations during the first trimester (or early in the second) will be how and when to tell your superiors and co-workers of your pregnancy. With most associates, of course, nothing need be said, but with supervisors and others whose work will be directly affected by your absence—temporary or permanent—notification is in order.

• *When you decide to make your pregnancy public, tell your immediate superior first.* Confiding in your luncheon partners first may be more rewarding, but your news is apt to become grist for the gossip mills. Gossip may reach your boss long before you do, thus undermining your relationship, raising questions about your commitment, and indicating a lack of trust. No matter how self-conscious and awkward you feel (and we all do!), it is *your* responsibility to notify your superiors. Don't depend on an intermediary.

• *Be smart about timing.* Some women are discreet about their pregnancies until they reach the fourth month, when the greatest likelihood of miscarriage is past. Besides, it is often a good idea for job-related reasons to hold off an announcement as long as possible. First, you give yourself more time if your company will want to know your future employment plans right away. Second, if you are being considered for a raise or promotion, pregnancy can be an obstacle. While it is discriminatory and a violation of federal law to deny a raise or promotion on the basis of pregnancy, it could be hard to prove that, for example, as *large* a raise as you felt you were entitled to was denied because of pregnancy.

If you think that a large raise or promotion is unimportant because you will be leaving work anyway, consider the future, when you might be reentering the job market as a $17,000 supervisor rather than a $15,000 assistant. Also, if a raise or promotion is scheduled for your ninth month, fight to get it, even if you won't have time to enjoy much of it.

Of course, some women think they owe their employers the earliest possible notification. This may be a legitimate feeling, but keep in mind the disadvantages.

• *Plan in advance the talk you will have with your supervisor.* Why are you telling your boss you are pregnant? To share the news? To work out time off for appointments with your doctor? To explain that you will be leaving after your seventh month? If you plan this conversation ahead of time, you may be able to limit the discussion to those issues you want to resolve. If you don't yet want to talk about how long you will work, or whether you'll be back after the baby's birth, don't bring up those topics. Unless you think things through first, you may find yourself making some commitments you're not really ready for.

Most women recommend forthrightness. You needn't—and shouldn't—be apologetic or embarrassed; nor should you overemphasize your condition. It is completely unnecessary to indicate that you'll continue to perform up to par. Also, figure out what your needs during pregnancy might be and make them known. For example, explain that you will occasionally need extra hours to accommodate monthly physician appointments. One woman commented, "Plenty of men visit doctors once a month, too!"

• *Avoid, as long as you can, any discussion of long-range plans.* (1) You adore your job; your salary is enviable; you are advancing steadily. You're certain you'll be back at your desk a month or two after the birth. (2) Your first three months of pregnancy have been a breeze. You're energetic and happy, and work is as enjoyable as ever. You know you'll work until you go into labor.

If you identify with (1) or (2), you may think it is reasonable, early on, to tell your plans to your employer. The fact is, you may change your mind. Many women do *not* stick to their original intentions. As you talk to other mothers, new options take shape, and as the baby grows, you may find your feelings changing, too.

. Working throughout pregnancy is certainly an economic benefit, but some first-time expectant mothers can't anticipate how fatigued they may feel during the last month, or how much time they will need to get things ready for the baby. On the other hand, your experience may be similar to one mother's, who recalled, "I *wish* I had worked during the last month. I got antsy. And of course my not working was a financial strain."

If co-workers ask about your future plans—and they will—be noncommittal. You might say, "I appreciate your interest. I just haven't made a decision yet."

As you feel better: the second trimester

As you reach the middle trimester, you probably feel better, your pregnancy is more familiar, and maternity clothes help you feel comfortable. You may have stopped pressuring yourself about how long to work and decided to take life one day at a time. Possibly you are looking at the future practically, thinking of part-time work and baby-sitting arrangements.

As your pregnancy becomes obvious to others, your relationship with co-workers may change. They may think of you more as a pregnant woman than as a lawyer or manager. If you pride yourself on professionalism, this shift can be frustrating. If your colleagues are mostly young and single, they may not take much interest in your pregnancy, or you may feel you cannot share your feelings. If you feel isolated or unsupported, it may be time to accept the divergence of interests gracefully. You may enjoy new acquaintances among those who are already parents.

It's not uncommon for a pregnant woman to feel she must prove herself: work twice as hard, stay late, drag herself to the job when ill—to show that she is the same professional she has always been. Said one employed mother: "I took no sick days, attended Lamaze classes evenings, and made doctor appointments on Saturdays. I thought it was important to set an example for skeptical men." A college teacher said, "I worked hard all the way—even dragged myself to class with the flu so I wouldn't be thought of as shirking."

It's hard *not* to pressure yourself—especially if your job is a responsible one. In the long run, though, you'll feel better if you make no more than the usual demands on yourself. Remember, no one expects you to work *harder* during pregnancy.

Getting comfortable on the job

•*Snacking.* Many women are surprised to find that their appetite increases when they are pregnant. They feel ravenous at 10:00 A.M. and again soon after lunch. If they are unprepared at work, they grab a candy bar. Obviously, you can do better for yourself and your baby by snacking nutritiously. Here are some convenient snacks pregnant women have enjoyed in the office:

raisins
carrot sticks, raw broccoli, and cauliflowerets—dip in plain
    yogurt mixed with dry salad

celery stuffed with cream cheese or peanut butter
cinnamon-dusted apple or pear slices
banana
hardboiled eggs and crackers
dried fruits mixed with nuts and shredded coconut
cheese hunks and tomato slices
small cans of fruit juice
Thermos filled with a milkshake
bouillon or instant soup
yogurt or cottage cheese; mix in fruit and vegetables
granola, dry cereals
baby-food-size jars of applesauce and puddings

Make a point of bringing a healthful snack every day. You'll
have more energy and be more alert.

• *Smoking.* You've given it up, but your co-workers haven't. If
they drift into your office while smoking, ask that they snuff out
cigarettes. The smoke is hazardous to you and to your baby.

• *Lunching.* At some offices, noontime is the social zenith and
lunch is not so much eaten as enjoyed. At other workplaces, lunch
is a bite on the run or a sandwich at the desk. No matter what kind
of lunch you're used to, be sure it is healthful. Don't ever skip the
midday meal. Take the full period you are permitted, and if you
finish early, take the extra time to rest or walk.

• *Lunch should be unrushed.* Keep shopping and running errands to a minimum, particularly during the last trimester when
you're apt to tire more easily. Chores can wait—eat lunch first.
Don't skip lunch when you go for your prenatal checkup.

• *Eat out or in?* Bringing a meal from home is a good idea if
lunch is apt to be a hot dog grabbed from a vendor. You can pack
something more nutritious. On the other hand, brown-baggers
who are tempted to lunch while working should set aside a little
time *just* for eating.

• *Eliminate social drinking.* The documented dangers to the fetus from alcohol suggest that you eliminate it entirely from your
diet now. Drinking may make you sleepy or less efficient, too, es-

pecially early in pregnancy. Take fruit juice instead and don't be apologetic.

Exercise

One of the more energizing things you can do when pregnant is to change position: lie down if you've been standing; walk if you've been sitting; stretch your spine and limbs. Unfortunately, office-bound workers have little opportunity to move, and this sedentary style can be uncomfortable during pregnancy. Try these suggestions:

• Do the pelvic rock while seated: three or four times, press your lower spine into the back of your chair until you feel tension released. Alternatively, try the pelvic rock while standing. Simply press the lower spine against door, wall, or the side of a file cabinet.

• Slide a box, upturned wastebasket, or stack of phone directories under your desk to prop up your feet.

• Choose a chair with a comfortable backrest. One that is too high will force you to arch your lower back; one that is too low will make you slump forward. If you sit at a typist's chair, the backrest should reach the small of your back. Armrests help support the torso and take some of the strain off back muscles. Remember that improper seating—or sitting for long hours—can aggravate varicose veins and hemorrhoids. Try not to cross your legs while sitting—this diminishes circulation.

• If you have a private office, try putting your legs up on a stool during the lunch hour and take a nap. Or lie on the carpeted floor on your left side for half an hour to reduce pressure on your lower extremities.

• Remove or loosen your shoes; flex, extend, and shake your feet; wiggle your toes; rotate your legs and feet; or push your feet against a wall to promote circulation in your legs. To relax your torso, try rotating your shoulders, head, and arms clockwise and counterclockwise; flex, extend, and shake your hands; massage the back of your neck. Make a morning and afternoon routine out of desk-side exercises, starting and ending each set with deep, relaxed breathing.

• Try counterpressure. Press your stockinged feet against the bar at the rear of your desk; push your hands or round your back against a wall or the door.

• Walk around the office while taking rhythmic, relaxed, deep breaths.

• When typing, don't hunch over the typewriter, but keep your back fairly straight. If you work at a high desk, sit on a stool with a back and use a footrest to keep your knees comfortably bent. In a conference room, don't sink into big, soft chairs; sit up straight. Whatever you do, be conscious of supporting, and thus relaxing, the small of your back.

The last months

The expectations you have of yourself, your physical condition, the kind of job and income you have, and your company's policy on leaves of absence will all contribute to your decision on how long to continue working outside the home during pregnancy. Many women enjoy working right up to delivery; they have few physical complaints and appreciate the money. Others prefer a hiatus between employment and baby care, a kind of "psychic breathing space." Don't permit other people to cajole or shame you either into staying or into quitting. Make your choice based on what you feel most comfortable doing.

If you do work through the last trimester, you may slow down as fatigue, awkwardness, and backache increase. It is especially important now to get plenty of sleep, to exercise, to eat well, and to nap when you can. If you find yourself coming in late and taking many days off, it might be time to consider a leave of absence or a resignation.

As in the first trimester, some women who plan to stay home after the baby's birth report feeling detached and less interested in work during the last weeks of pregnancy. It's almost as if they have less psychic energy to spread around as motherhood becomes imminent. They know they are leaving work, and they may become withdrawn from colleagues and issues that will still be there after they have gone. Adding to the withdrawal process is the guilt some women feel about slowing down.

If you are experiencing this detachment and focusing more and more on your baby, it may be time to leave work if you can manage the finances and know you won't be bored.

If you plan to return to work after the birth, you may not feel so withdrawn, but you may have ambivalent feelings if you've been fielding disparaging comments about mothers who work. As you arrange your leave, try to take as much of it as possible after the birth so that you have a solid block of time to become acquainted with your child. But give yourself some time, too, before the baby is born for rest and relaxation. Although you may be under pressure to make arrangements for the weeks you will be gone, resist the temptation to stay late or work on weekends. Consider how exhausted you would be if you went into labor after ten hours of work.

Comments from pregnant working women:

"Even though I lost time [teaching at a college] before and after the baby's birth, my employer was amply compensated in terms of hard work both before and after the birth."

"Take catnaps at your desk and ask your secretary to buzz you after ten minutes."

"I am very tired but feel that staying home wouldn't be healthy."

"Working outside the home while I was pregnant was less tiring than caring for toddlers while pregnant."

"Good shoes and support hose if you're a nurse!"

"My employer wasn't too pleased, but my hours had to be altered because after three P.M. I was so exhausted that I wasn't up to par. I started leaving work early. After my sixth month I quit."

"If you work up to the last minute, and don't have the opportunity to meet other stay-at-home mothers, you might be very lonely after the baby is born and you are home alone."

"I taught and had a problem with nausea. It helped to keep raisins in my desk for discreet snacking. Also, I chose an obstetrician who could schedule appointments late in the day."

"I intended to go back to work in six weeks, but after three weeks postpartum, I couldn't bear to leave my son. Naturally, this disappointed a lot of people and botched their planning."

From a law student: "I stood out in class because I was pregnant. My professors took a special interest in me."

"Don't be ashamed—you're no superwoman!"

"I took sick leave an hour at a time for doctor appointments."

"I felt exhilarated and energized! I never worked better!"

"I asked others not to smoke in my office."

"I wish I had quit months ahead. I was exhausted and depressed. Although I had performed my job well, I was pretty insufferable at home."

Is your job safe?

According to the American College of Obstetricians and Gynecologists' booklet *Guidelines on Pregnancy and Work:* "The normal woman with an uncomplicated pregnancy and a normal fetus in a job that presents no greater potential hazards than those encountered in normal daily life in the community may continue to work without interruption until the onset of labor. . . ." In other words, if you and the baby are healthy and your job poses no dangers, you can safely work as long as you wish.

You and your obstetrician can make determinations about your health and your baby's. But what are the dangers—sometimes unseen or unrecognized—that a job may pose?

• *Operational*. Pushing, stretching, lifting, pulling, constant sitting or standing, or other activities that may be hazardous to you or uncomfortable when you are pregnant.

• *Chemical.* Substances that you inhale, touch, or swallow when pregnant that may be teratogenic or may impair the mother's system in such a way that the fetus suffers or dies.

• *Environmental.* Extremes in humidity or temperature that can cause significant discomfort to pregnant women; or loud noise or vibration, which some research studies indicate may be harmful to the fetus over long periods of time.

• *Infectious diseases.* Hospital personnel, women doing biological research involving infectious organisms, and teachers of young children risk frequent exposure to some diseases that cause congenital malformations, abortion, or fetal distress.

• *Ionizing radiation.* Exposure in medical or industrial settings that may cause malformations or cancer in the unborn child.

Operational hazards

If you have been employed for some time at a job requiring physical labor, pregnancy may not alter your ability to work. Your body may be so familiar with the demands placed upon it that you can perform your job with ease.

Many women, however, particularly during the last trimester, find lifting loads, extensive climbing, and any task that requires good balance, difficult and possibly dangerous. A protruding abdomen requires not only that you reposition what you carry but also that you employ muscles you may not be accustomed to using to lift and to maintain your balance. Back muscles feel the new strains, and already stretched pelvic ligaments can make twisting painful.

Women who work at a desk are not immune to operational difficulties. If they cannot move about, find comfortable seating, or adjust working hours to make commuting less taxing, they, too, will suffer fatigue, muscular strain, and loss of appetite. Women who stand all day—salespeople, guides, and cashiers, for example—are vulnerable to varicose veins, hemorrhoids, fatigue, and strain.

Chemical hazards

The fetus is extraordinarily sensitive to chemical influences. Its rapidly dividing cells can easily be harmed. Abortion and malformation may result from toxic contacts, or a fetus may grow to become a maimed or cancer-susceptible adult. Learning disabilities and personality disturbances can result from toxic exposure.

In a 1976 Conference on Women and the Workplace, sponsored by the Society for Occupational and Environmental Health, Dr. Shirley Conibear called fetuses "exquisitely sensitive to any lack of necessary nutrients or blockage of their use. Any disruption in cell division, differentiation or migration is irreversible and is magnified thousands of times in the adult."

We now know that, contrary to popular belief, the placenta does *not* screen out all harmful substances. One medical writer described the placenta as a sieve. Almost all chemicals—toxic or not—can pass from mother to infant.

According to the ACOG's booklet *Guidelines,* the following chemicals have been associated with hazards to the fetus or to the reproductive systems of male and female animals and/or men and women:

- heavy metals: cadmium; lead; mercury
- organic solvents: benzene (benzol)
- halogenated hydrocarbons: 2 chlorobutadiene (chloroprene); dibromochloropropane; epichlorohydrin; ethylene dibromide; polychlorinated biphenyls (PCBs); tetrachloroethylene (perchloroethylene); vinyl chloride
- hypoxic agents: carbon monoxide
- anesthetic gases: halogenated gases
- pesticides: carbaryl, chlorinated hydrocarbons; chlordecone (kepone)
- miscellaneous: carbon disulfide; ethylene oxide

A chemical sampler

Some of the above chemicals are clearly linked to fetal harm. Through tragic experience or testing, we know what damage they can cause. A few specifics:

• *Lead.* For centuries it has been known that excessive lead ingestion can cause sterility; some historians even believe the widespread use of lead pots may have caused the dying out of Rome's upper classes, leading to the fall of the Roman Empire. Today, we know that lead can affect the central nervous system, kidneys, and blood-forming organs, and that it can cross the placenta and have grave affects on the fetus. The high rate of abortions and stillbirths among female workers exposed to high lead levels, the susceptibility of their newborns to convulsions, and the high concentrations of lead in the placenta, liver, and brain of some lead workers' stillborn infants indicate the hazards. It is also believed that excessive lead levels cause birth defects, prematurity, and infant mortality.

According to Dr. Kenneth Bridbord of the National Institute of Occupational Safety and Health, people who work with lead frequently breathe air contaminated with quantities of the metal a hundred to a thousand times greater than that in normal air; workers may take in lead from contaminated fingers, lips, cigarettes, and clothes. Organolead compounds, used as gasoline additives, may be absorbed through the skin. Dr. Sidney Lerner, of the Department of Environmental Health of the University of Cincinnati, said to the Conference on Women and the Workplace: ". . . it has been my recommendation to persons responsible for the health of lead workers that fertile, gravid, or nursing females not be employed in areas where there will be increased lead exposure, albeit safe for the workers, until such time as adequate information has been developed proving the safety of such exposure to the fetus."

• *Mercury.* One of the great tragedies of the industrial age involved organic mercury: a petrochemical plant, for years discharging its wastes into Minamata Bay, Japan, not only poisoned the fish and the water but also brutally injured hundreds of residents of the area who consumed that fish. Pregnant women who ate the poisoned fish transmitted the mercury to their offspring. These babies grew up with problems ranging from mental deficiency to severe retardation, motor and sensory disturbances, seizures, deformities, and personality disturbances. Organic mercury compounds occur in agricultural and industrial production. Because of the tragic experiences at Minamata, scientists are certain of the effects mercury has on embryos and fetuses.

Although the effects of inorganic mercury are not so clear, we know that this form of mercury can also cross the placenta. Women who are likely to come in contact with this substance are dental assistants and dentists who breathe in the vapors as they prepare mercury amalgams.

• *Vinyl chloride.* This is a crucial compound in the plastics industry. Some studies have shown that vinyl chloride induces tumors in the offspring of exposed pregnant rats, and other researchers suggest there may be a link between vinyl chloride exposure in the mother and central nervous system defects in the offspring, as well as miscarriage and stillbirth. Perhaps the most significant cause of VC-related defects is exposure of the *father* to this toxic chemical. Vinyl chloride is necessary to the manufacture of *poly*vinyl chloride, which is molded into thousands of products, including construction materials, phonograph records, furniture, automobiles, fabric finishes, tubing, food packaging, bottles, toys, and appliances. Environmental scientist Dr. Samuel Epstein estimates that hundreds of thousands of employees work with VC or PVC.

• *Phthalic acid esters (PAEs).* Chemicals that give pliability to polyvinyl chloride containers also have been linked to birth defects in laboratory animals.

• *Anesthetic gases.* In 1971, researchers in California reported a study showing a 38 percent miscarriage rate among nurse-anesthetists as compared to a 10 percent rate among general-duty nurses. In many other countries as well, studies confirmed that operating-room personnel are at high risk during pregnancy—at risk of spontaneous abortion or of bearing a child with congenital defects. The cause is thought to be the waste anesthetic gases that escape into the air during surgical procedures. Some researchers believe that even the wives of male operating-room personnel are at risk.

• *PCBs.* In 1968, a strange disease broke out in Japan. Infants were born with dark-brown-tinted skin. The "cola-colored" babies were small, showing intrauterine growth retardation. The cause was eventually traced to a certain brand of rice cooking oil. It was found to be contaminated with polychlorinated biphenyls. PCBs are a global problem because traces of this compound have been found in the oceans, as well as in lakes, rivers, fish, and human tissue. Used primarily as coolants, but also, before 1971, found in plastics, paints, varnishes, and "carbonless" carbon paper, these toxic chemicals are not biodegradable. They linger in our environment and bodies for generations.

These chemicals are but a partial listing. According to the Occupational Safety and Health Administration, there are more than twenty-five thousand identified toxic substances in the environment. Most of these and thousands more are untested for their effects on the fetus. Many may be teratogens, mutagens, transplacental carcinogens (capable of crossing the placenta to cause cancer in the offspring many years later), or abortifacients. We know, too, that sometimes chemicals can interact *synergistically*—that is, they can combine to create effects far worse than any one chemical alone could create. Scientists are far from pinpointing the synergistic reactions that can damage a fetus.

Pregnant women who work with toxic substances may touch them directly or may carry the substance on their garments. Toxic substances may be accidentally swallowed if a worker eats near the area where the material is handled. If a substance is in the air where everyone inhales it, a pregnant worker may be at greater risk than fellow workers. Because of changes in breathing patterns, women actually take in more air when they are pregnant. Thus, if a toxic substance is in the air, it will be inhaled in greater quantities by a pregnant woman.

If you have a desk job, you, too, may be at risk. Where is your desk located with reference to hazardous materials in the factory? To storage or dumping areas? Could poisonous substances permeate the air you breathe? Do you visit industrial areas where toxic substances are manufactured? Do you frequently walk through hazardous areas with no protection for your face or body? Do you handle office materials or machines that may contain toxic substances? It is vital that you become aware of your working environment. If you don't know the answers to these questions, it's important to find out.

The accompanying Table 3, reprinted from *Guidelines on Pregnancy and Work*, lists some occupations and associated toxic chemicals.

Table 3.
OCCUPATIONS AND ASSOCIATED TOXIC CHEMICALS

OCCUPATION

EXPOSURES

1. Textile and Related Operatives

  a. Textile operatives — raw cotton dust, noise, synthetic fiber dusts, formaldehyde, heat, dyes, flame retardants, asbestos

  b. Sewers and stitchers — cotton and synthetic fiber dusts, noise, formaldehyde, organic solvents, flame retardants, asbestos

  c. Upholsterers — same as above

(Some specific chemicals encountered in the above occupations are: benzene, toluene, trichloroethylene, perchloroethylene, chloroprene, styrene, carbon disulfide.)

2. Hospital/Health Personnel

  a. Registered nurses, aides, orderlies — anesthetic gases, ethylene oxide, X-ray radiation, alcohol, infectious diseases, puncture wounds

  b. Dental hygienists — X-ray radiation, mercury, ultrasonic noise, anesthetic gases

  c. Laboratory workers (clinical and research) — wide variety of toxic chemicals, including carcinogens, mutagens, and teratogens, X-ray radiation

3. Electronics assemblers — lead, tin, antimony, trichloroethylene, methylene chloride, epoxy resins, methyl ethyl ketone

4. Hairdressers and cosmetologists — hair spray resins (polyvinyl pyrrolidone), aerosol propellants (freons), halogenated hydrocarbons, hair dyes, solvents of nail polish, benzyl alcohol, ethyl alcohol, acetone

OCCUPATION	EXPOSURES
5. Cleaning Personnel	
a. Launderers	soaps, detergents, enzymes, heat, humidity, industrially contaminated clothing
b. Dry cleaners	perchloroethylene, trichloroethylene, stoddard solvent (naphtha), benzene, industrially contaminated clothing
6. Photographic processors	caustics, iron salts, mercuric chloride, bromides, iodides, pyrogallic acid, and silver nitrate
7. Plastics fabricators	acrylonitrile, phenol-formaldehydes, urea-formaldehydes, hexamethylenetetramine, acids, alkalies, peroxide, vinyl chloride, polystyrene, vinylidene chloride
8. Domestics	solvents, hydrocarbons, soaps, detergents, bleaches, alkalies
9. Transportation operatives	carbon monoxide, polynuclear aromatics, lead, and other combustion products of gasoline, vibration, physical stresses
10. Sign painters and letterers	lead oxide, lead chromate pigments, epichlorohydrin, titanium dioxide, trace metals, xylene, toluene
11. Clerical personnel	physical stresses, poor illumination, trichloroethylene, carbon tetrachloride and various other cleaners, asbestos in air conditioning
12. Opticians and lens grinders	coal-tar pitch volatiles, iron oxide dust solvents, hydrocarbons
13. Printing operatives	ink mists, 2-nitropropane, methanol, carbon tetrachloride, methylene chloride, lead, noise, hydrocarbon solvents, trichloroethylene, toluene, benzene, trace metals

A word about fathers

Any discussion of women's work hazards would be incomplete without emphasizing that men may also be exposed to substances that can damage their unborn children. Some chemicals may affect sperm production so that fertilization may not be accomplished, or when fertilization does take place, the father's damaged germ cell may cause malformation in the embryo. Abortion may result. Vinyl chloride, lead, kepone, mercury, cadmium, and dibromochloropropane are substances known to be potentially damaging to *fathers*, and it's becoming clear to researchers concerned with the unborn that workplaces must be made safe not only for women but also for men.

Environmental hazards

During pregnancy, when a woman's physiology is working to get rid of her baby's body heat as well as her own, excess environmental heat can be stressful. Physically demanding work in a hot environment makes heat release from the body even more difficult. If the air is humid, the body will have difficulty cooling because sweat will take longer to evaporate. The results may be fainting, dizziness, or drowsiness—all of which may be dangerous if a woman is working with machinery or is driving, or when she must depend on balance or speed to perform. Heat may be so stressful that heatstroke can result.

Women who work in the presence of loud, continuous noise may also be putting their babies at risk. A California study linked noise at Los Angeles County Airport to the high rate of birth defects found in newborns whose mothers lived near the airport. The defects included cleft palate, harelip, and damage to the brain, spinal cord, and abdomen. Although these findings have been disputed, we *do* know that noise can cause irritability, stimulate the release of adrenaline, and contract blood vessels. Researchers theorize that these reactions can cause oxygen to be denied to the fetus.

Infectious diseases

In some professions, contact with disease is an occupational hazard. Teachers of small children frequently see German measles, flu, and chicken pox; hospital personnel are exposed to hepatitis and other viral infections. Laboratory workers—clinical or research—handle a variety of cultures of infectious diseases. Should a pregnant worker be exposed, the problem could be serious. Infection places an extra burden on the pregnant body, and recovery can be slow and uncomfortable. Some ordinarily prescribed drugs may be contraindicated. Finally, and most important, some viral infections in the mother cause abortion, deformities, or disease in the fetus. These include rubella (German measles), measles, mumps, herpes zoster and herpes simplex, influenza (A-strain), lymphocytic choriomeningitis, cytomegalic inclusion, hepatitis A (infectious), anterior poliomyelitis, Coxsackie virus, smallpox, and chicken pox.

Diseases not caused by viruses, including toxoplasmosis and syphilis, are also dangerous to the fetus.

If you work in a job that increases your chances of exposure to viral disease, find out which diseases can be prevented by vaccination. It's a good idea to be inoculated *before* you begin a pregnancy.

Ionizing radiation

The dangers of radiation to the fetus from diagnostic X rays have been discussed in Chapter 5. Pregnant women who work in jobs that may entail exposure to harmful radiation put their babies at risk without a concomitant medical benefit. These workers include nuclear medicine and X-ray technicians, nurses, physicians, dental assistants, dentists, laboratory workers, nuclear reactor workers, and nuclear technologists. Some researchers have suggested that flight attendants may be exposed to harmful radiation from poorly shielded radioactive materials in the cargo holds of airplanes.

Workers whose jobs involve radiation exposure often wear film badges or other personal dosimeters to show the amounts of radiation the employee has absorbed. Dose levels are recorded, and workers have a legal right to obtain their records. Women who expect to be pregnant should know their monthly dose levels and report this information to their physicians. They should speak with their union representatives about job hazards. If they go to their company's health officer—and this may be necessary—they may be advised to quit, accept a transfer, or take a leave of absence, or they may be fired. Although these options are unfair and discriminatory, they may be the only choices women have.

The National Council on Radiation Protection and Measurement recommends a total fetal dose—through the nine-month period of pregnancy—of 0.5 rem (*r*oentgen *e*quivalent *m*an). For comparison, it helps to know that the average dose from a chest X ray is 0.045 rem, and that natural background radiation for all of us averages 0.13 rem a year. The nuclear accident at Three Mile Island in Pennsylvania in 1979 exposed nearby residents to 0.08 rem, according to experts.

What to do about job hazards

It is one thing to know or experience problems on the job because of your pregnancy and quite another to cope with them. If a job is physically demanding, you may quit early in pregnancy, losing seniority, maternity-leave benefits, and any possibility of reentry. Some women delay notifying their employers about their pregnancy because they are afraid they will immediately be fired, demoted, or transferred to a lower-paying job the employer deems safer (although these actions *may* be illegal—see Chapter 15).

The consequences of delay can be tragic if chemicals or radiation are damaging the infant all the while. At the same time, a woman dependent on her livelihood may fear the immediate loss of income more than an ill-defined future threat to her child. While no woman should have to make a choice between livelihood and pregnancy, that is precisely the situation many expectant mothers face.

Laws are not clear when it comes to the thorny questions of pregnant women in hazardous occupations, although laws do exist that guarantee both a safe working environment and equal employment opportunity. A 1978 amendment to the 1964 Civil Rights Act forbids discrimination on the basis of pregnancy. The Occupational Safety and Health Administration's director, Dr. Eula Bingham, says OSHA's commitment is to protection of all workers, and warns that employers who single out certain kinds of workers and exclude them, instead of making the working environment safe, may be violating the law.

Yet it seems that there are situations in which the working environment simply cannot be made safe for a fetus. Increasingly, too, employers fear the possibility that a person deformed *in utero* will sue them. Many large companies say, too, that the cost of making the working environment safe for pregnant women would be prohibitive or that they simply do not know what constitutes a "safe environment" for such employees. They ask women employees to submit proof of sterility or to undergo pregnancy tests in order to work in certain jobs. They may fire, transfer, or demote pregnant women or ask them to take a leave of absence.

Apparently, such exclusions may be legal when the employer has tried but found it impossible to make the workplace safe. The

Equal Employment Opportunity Commission warns, however: "Exclusionary employment actions taken hastily or without regard for rigorous adherence to acceptable scientific processes may be viewed as unlawful discrimination." OSHA stresses that employers should consider job rotation, transfer, and rate retention—having the employee keep the same pay, benefits, and seniority when transferred—before resorting to firing.

Safe for everybody

Some women's advocates declare that any double standard is discriminatory. They point out that there are virtually no corporate policies regarding male reproduction, which can also be affected by toxic substances, and that there should not be multiple safety standards, there should be only one—for human beings, including men, women, and fetuses.

Many researchers wonder about substances found unsafe for fetuses. Might not these compounds then be unsafe for all living things? Is it not an instance of discrimination against *men* if they are permitted to work with toxic substances? And most people seem to agree with OSHA that if a workplace cannot be made safe for pregnant workers, those workers should be transferred to safer areas with no loss of seniority, benefits, or salary.

The Occupational Safety and Health Act of 1970 was enacted "to assure so far as possible every working man and woman in the nation safe and healthful working conditions, and to preserve our human resources." OSHA sets safe exposure levels for many toxic substances. Many trade organizations, unions, and large corporations have done their own studies and formulated guidelines about safety in the workplace. The information is available, even though its impact may be hotly debated.

If your work brings you close to substances of questionable safety (questionable in *your* mind), be sure to find out what, exactly, those substances are, so that you can notify your physician. In some cases, employers regularly monitor exposure levels and make these data available. In other cases, you may be better off contacting your union. Sometimes information about toxic substances will be extremely difficult to obtain. Your employer may refer you to a supplier, who may in turn refer you to another supplier. Ingredients may be considered trade secrets and thus may not be available to the public. (However, OSHA may be able to determine the hazards of secret ingredients.) Materials may bear trade names that give no clue to their components.

As a worker, however, you do have rights. According to an OSHA booklet, these include:

- the right to review copies of any OSHA rules and standards that your employer is required to make available at the workplace
- the right to request information from your employer on safety and health hazards in the area and on precautions taken against these hazards
- the right to request, in writing, that the OSHA area director conduct an investigation of your working environment (if you do exercise this right, be prepared to specify the potential hazard)
- the right to have your name withheld from your employer when you request an OSHA inspection
- the right to file a complaint with OSHA if you believe you have been discriminated against for asserting the above rights

If you or your physician needs more information about toxic substances and their effects, you may tap a variety of sources:

1. *The Occupational Safety and Health Administration, 200 Constitution Avenue, N.W., Washington, D.C. 20210,* investigates complaints and sets and enforces standards for healthful working environments. OSHA representatives will conduct inspections of workplaces, and OSHA also publishes fact sheets on standards, hazards, and regulations. There are ten regional offices and about a hundred area offices. Look for the address of the office nearest you in the telephone directory under United States Government—Labor Department.

2. *The National Institute of Occupational Safety and Health, Parklawn Building, 5600 Fishers Lane, Rockville, MD 20857,* is the principal federal agency doing research on occupational hazards. NIOSH also investigates workplaces and recommends standards of safety. If you (or your physician) have a question about the safety of your job, NIOSH's researchers, physicians, and industrial hygienists can get you information. NIOSH also publishes the *Registry of Toxic Effects of Chemical Substances,* which contains a wealth of information on various compounds and can be found in many university libraries. (A lay person may have difficulty deciphering the data, however.) NIOSH has ten regional offices. Look in your telephone directory under United States Government—Department of Health, Education, and Welfare.

3. *American College of Obstetricians and Gynecologists, 1 East Wacker Drive, Chicago, IL 60601,* publishes *Guidelines on Pregnancy and Work*

and an accompanying bibliography. Your physician can obtain copies from the ACOG, and can also obtain research data on specific hazards. Lay people who call or write (to the Resource Center at the same address) may receive literature or be referred to a hospital, public interest group, or physician in their area who can help with occupational health questions.

4. *Local committees.* Your state or city may have a public interest group or coalition of unions committed to occupational safety and health. A local university or hospital may have specialists in the area.

5. *State or city governments* may have occupational safety and health departments, partially funded by OSHA, with rules and standards at least as strict as OSHA's. Such departments may offer inspections, research material, and publications.

6. *Your union* may have special guidelines for pregnant women and will help you with the serious problem of discrimination. It will let you know about contractual provisions that affect pregnant workers.

7. *Women's Occupational Health Resource Center, American Health Foundation, 320 East 43rd Street, New York, NY 10017,* has a computerized library service, fact sheets, bulletins, and a working woman's newsletter.

CHAPTER FIFTEEN
Your Job Rights

Traditionally, pregnant women have been targets for discriminatory employment practices. Many employers used to feel—and some still do—that pregnancy always hampers work performance and interferes with the efficient operation of a business. In the past, women who wanted to work during pregnancy were often fired, forced to take maternity leave, or denied benefits offered to other disabled workers. But a 1978 amendment to Title VII of the 1964 Civil Rights Act specifically makes it unlawful for employers to discriminate against pregnant women.

The amendment became law on October 31, 1978. It applies to employers of fifteen or more people, and to employers of any size who do business with the federal government. The amendment makes it clear that:

1. A woman's job status cannot suffer just because she's pregnant.

2. Pregnancy must be treated as any other temporary disability is treated under "fringe benefit programs," such as sick leave, medical and hospital insurance, and disability insurance.

The amendment does not mean that pregnant women will be treated better than other workers, or receive benefits others do not. The law merely ensures equal treatment for the pregnant employee, based on her ability or inability to work. It should also be noted that a pregnant woman need not be married to enjoy the rights and benefits provided by the amendment. Job issues affected by the new amendment include the following.

Hiring, training, promoting

The 1978 amendment reemphasizes what earlier federal guidelines said: *an employer cannot refuse to hire a woman simply because she's pregnant.* In fact, an employer cannot ask a prospective employee if she is pregnant or plans to be, unless the employer asks every applicant about anticipated temporary disabilities. In that case, though, the information about pregnancy could not be used as a basis for not hiring the applicant.

An employer cannot use the fact a worker is pregnant to bar her from promotion or additional training. In the past, women were frequently kept in low-paying, low-prestige jobs because their employers did not want to promote workers who were "just going to get pregnant, anyway." Also, pregnant workers were often denied promotions and extra training—and thus the salary increases that came with them—because employers assumed they would be leaving soon and would probably not be returning. The amendment makes it clear that such unequal treatment is unlawful.

For planning purposes, *an employer can require that an employee report her pregnancy as soon as it's confirmed.* But again, this practice is lawful only when the employer requires all employees to report conditions that may temporarily prevent them from working.

Dismissal

A worker cannot be fired just because she is pregnant, as long as she is able to work. If a pregnant employee is not performing up to par, she may be treated as any other worker would be, whether that means dismissal, enforced leave of absence, or transfer to a less demanding position.

Leaves of absence

Over the years, employers have recognized that pregnancy and childbirth might temporarily prevent women from working. So some offered "maternity leave," usually a fixed amount of time off without pay, after which the employee could return with no loss in position, salary, or benefits. Depending on the employer, this period ranged from several weeks to two years.

Under the 1978 amendment to the Civil Rights Act, *maternity leave is no longer distinct from medical leave for other temporary disabilities.* This means that a pregnant woman cannot be forced on leave when she is still capable of working, or be forced to stay on leave for a certain length of time, or be recalled after a set period when other disabled employees are not subject to the same treatment.

An employer cannot demand to know in advance if and when a pregnant employee will be taking or returning from medical leave unless other workers who will be temporarily disabled must report such information. On the other hand, pregnant women cannot be fired for *taking* a medical leave unless the employer's policy is to fire all temporarily disabled workers. (Some state laws provide that a pregnant woman *must* be given a reasonable amount of time for medical leave, even when her employer has no policy regarding such leave. Union contracts often guarantee leaves of absence for pregnancy and childbirth, also.)

Some employers may require a doctor's certification before allowing a pregnant woman to continue working, or before allowing her to return from medical leave. This procedure is lawful, provided workers with other medical conditions or on medical leave are treated in the same way. For example, an employer may want to be sure a heart-attack victim returning to work can handle his old job, and so may require a doctor's okay. The employer can even require a pregnant woman to be examined by the company doctor if that is the policy for other workers.

A woman returning from medical leave for pregnancy and childbirth cannot be asked about her child-care arrangements unless other temporarily disabled workers must provide this information.

Transfer

An employer cannot transfer a pregnant employee to an easier job on the assumption she will be unable to handle her regular work. However, if the fetus may be harmed by certain substances in the working environment, the employer may have sufficient legal grounds for the transfer. On the other hand, pregnant women who *are* having difficulty with their work may be able to arrange such a transfer—either directly with their employers or through a union contract—instead of going on medical leave.

Medical benefits

Many companies and organizations offer health insurance plans to help employees pay their medical and hospital bills. The terms and conditions of the insurance are decided by the employer and the insurance company offering the coverage. *The 1978 amendment affects these health insurance plans by requiring that pregnancy, child-*

birth, and related conditions be treated in the same way as other medical conditions. (Abortion—except to save the mother's life—is specifically excluded from this portion of the amendment's coverage.)

Employers cannot attach special conditions to pregnancy coverage, such as a time period before coverage becomes effective, unless other medical conditions are dealt with similarly in the insurance plan. Again, the amendment does not mean pregnancy will be treated preferentially. Employers are not required to set up health insurance plans if they have none, or to offer greater coverage for pregnancy than for other medical conditions.

Disability benefits

Many employers provide their workers with some compensation when they are temporarily unable to work. Employees may get *sick leave*—usually a certain number of days off with pay that are allowed for illness each year. If an employee is disabled for longer periods of time, the employer may provide *disability insurance,* which will pay part or all of the worker's wages for a set period (often eight, thirteen, twenty-six, or fifty-two weeks).

Under the 1978 amendment, pregnancy cannot be treated differently from other disabilities when it comes to benefits such as sick leave or disability insurance. A woman who cannot work because of pregnancy or childbirth is entitled to the same amount of paid and/or unpaid sick leave as other disabled workers. When an employee wants time off during pregnancy although not actually disabled, she will probably have to arrange for *personal leave,* which is often unpaid. If during personal leave a woman becomes disabled by her pregnancy, she may be able to convert the personal leave to sick leave, but this will depend on how her employer handles similar situations.

As is the case with health insurance plans, employers cannot exclude pregnancy from disability insurance plans in which other temporary disabilities are covered.

Seniority and reinstatement

In 1977 the U.S. Supreme Court ruled that a worker returning from maternity leave cannot be stripped of the seniority she earned prior to taking the leave. The 1978 amendment reaffirms this decision. *No woman will lose her job status or benefits merely because she was pregnant.*

A woman returning from medical leave for pregnancy and childbirth must also be reinstated in the same way other employees returning from medical leave are reinstated. For some workers this means returning to the same job they left. For others, it means assuming a new position, but one equivalent in status and pay to their previous one.

Unemployment benefits

Unemployment insurance is a program set up by the government and funded in part by private employers. The program provides compensation for workers who become unemployed through no fault of their own and are looking for another job. Although the federal government originally authorized the unemployment insurance program, each state has specific laws governing those who are eligible for compensation, how much they can receive, and when they can begin to receive it.

The 1978 amendment eliminates pregnancy as a reason to seek compensation—simply because termination on the basis of pregnancy is now illegal. However, a woman may lose her job during pregnancy for reasons other than her condition, such as business closings or job cutbacks. In those cases, she is entitled to collect unemployment compensation just like any other worker, provided she makes herself available for work. If a woman voluntarily leaves her job during pregnancy or because of it, she may have difficulty collecting compensation, but this decision is subject to individual state law. For information about unemployment compensation, contact your state unemployment insurance office, which is often a division of your state department of labor.

Discrimination and what to do about it

The 1978 amendment does not mean discriminatory practices against women will become nonexistent. But if a working woman feels she's subject to discrimination because of her pregnancy and cannot resolve the matter with her employer, she has recourse to:

•*Equal Employment Opportunity Commission (EEOC).* The EEOC is the federal agency set up to investigate complaints of Title VII violations. If the EEOC finds a complaint is justified, it will first try to resolve the problem by talking with the employer and the employee. If these efforts fail, the commission will either (1) bring suit against the employer in federal court or (2) issue a "right-to-sue" letter allowing the employee to bring suit in federal court. If the EEOC does not issue a right-to-sue letter, the employee may request the letter, then bring suit herself within ninety days.

• *State agencies.* Besides federal laws, all states have some anti-discrimination laws administered by such agencies as the state fair employment practices commission or human rights commission. In some cases, state laws are more liberal than federal laws and provide added protection for pregnant workers.

• *Local agencies.* Some municipalities have set up their own commissions to investigate complaints of discrimination in employment.

• *Office of Federal Contract Compliance Programs (OFCCP).* This federal agency enforces executive orders that prohibit companies doing business with the federal government from discriminating against employees and applicants because of race, color, religion, national origin, or sex.

• *Unions.* Most collective-bargaining agreements include an antidiscrimination clause. Women should follow their union's grievance procedures to report pregnancy discrimination and have it stopped.

• *Women's groups.* Some working women may not be protected by Title VII (because they work for employers of fewer than fifteen people), by state laws (which may also have numerical restrictions), or by union contract. Such workers could get help by contacting a local or national women's group. These groups may be able to influence the employers to halt discriminatory practices.

Business necessity

As we've mentioned, the 1978 amendment does not mean pregnant working women will never face job discrimination. However, employers will have to show that they did not discriminate against a worker solely because of her pregnancy.

To explain discriminatory actions, an employer may use the "business necessity" defense. That is, the employer may claim that a pregnant employee's termination (or leave, or transfer, or whatever) was essential to the safe and efficient operation of the business. For example, in the past, airlines have defended in court their policy of mandatory maternity leave by showing that passenger safety might be hampered by pregnant flight attendants.

Business necessity may also be asserted when a pregnant woman is transferred, terminated, or put on leave because her work environment may be hazardous to the fetus. In this case, the employer's first responsibility is to try to make the workplace safe for pregnant employees. However, laws are unclear as to how far an employer must go to accomplish this end. It is arguable that discriminatory actions are legal if after careful trial the employer has found it impossible to rid the environment of conditions hazardous to fetal health.

In any case, business necessity is very difficult to prove. Moreover, the law says that even when business necessity indicates discrimination may be justified, the employer must perform the least discriminatory act possible—for example, transfer rather than leave, or leave rather than termination.

CHAPTER SIXTEEN
You *Can* Understand Your Insurance

Nobody likes to hang a price tag on a baby. Presumably, all it takes to have one is love, pride, and joy. But besides these intangibles you'll need a couple of thousand dollars in cold cash.

It is never too early in a pregnancy to begin financial planning for the birth. Even if you have health insurance, it is important that you examine your coverage early to see which charges are your responsibility and which are not. In this way, you can budget for your needs. Too many couples reach the eleventh hour, only to be shocked by the extensive charges *not* covered by insurance.

Maternity costs

The maternity financial picture is a jigsaw puzzle, with lots of pieces *you* have to fit together to determine your costs. In chronological sequence, the major charges you are likely to incur include:

• *Obstetrician.* Usually a lump-sum fee charged by the physician by the time of birth. It covers prenatal care, labor and delivery, and postpartum checkups.

• *Prenatal tests.* Starting with your initial $15 pregnancy test, you may also have to budget for exams ranging from, say, a $25 blood series to a $75 ultrasound scan. These tests are *not* included in the obstetrician's fee.

• *Hospital.* Includes labor- and delivery-room charges, room and board for about three days, medications, special tests such as a predelivery X-ray pelvimetry or fetal monitoring, and nursery care for the infant.

•*Anesthesiologist.* Not included in the hospital charge unless s/he is an employee of the hospital.

•*Pediatrician.* A pediatrician visits the baby during your hospital stay.

Hospital costs

In mid-1978, the Health Insurance Institute surveyed more than thirty hospitals across the country to determine maternity costs. The institute found that the average hospital stay was 3.3 days. On this basis, they computed the following costs for labor and delivery and postpartum stay:

Room and board—3.3 days at $102 a day $336.60
Nursery—3.3 days at $66 a day 217.80
Labor room 79.00
Delivery room 153.00
Circumcision setup 10.00
Pharmacy (mother and baby) 39.00
Laboratory (mother and baby) 53.00
　　Total hospital charge $888.40

Doctors' fees

You must add physicians' fees to this figure. Yes, physicians—for there are several who attend you during pregnancy and birth. The average costs are as follows, according to 1977 statistics of the Health Insurance Association of America and *Medical Economics:*

Attending physician's complete obstetrical charge $351.00
Circumcision (performed by obstetrician) 29.00
Anesthesiologist 100–150.00
Pediatrician's newborn care 38.00
　　Total physicians' fees $518–568.00

Adding hospital charges to physicians' fees gives you the average total for medical care during pregnancy: $1,406.40 to 1,456.40. But remember, these are nationwide averages. If you opt to deliver at a major university-affiliated hospital, if you select specialists instead of general practitioners, and if you live in a large city, don't be surprised if your total costs exceed $2,000. For example, your room may cost $225 a day; the delivery room may cost $250. Even daily nursery charges may be $100 a day.

Women who have cesarean births—and they comprise at least 10 percent of us—may also be amazed at how expensive birth can be. A seven-day hospital stay may cost close to $1,000; seven-day nursery charges and more medication than is needed for a vaginal birth can push hospital charges higher. Your obstetrician will charge an extra $100 to $200 for the surgery; another surgeon may assist (you'll have to pay her/him, too); and anesthesia, of course, is not optional. The total bill for a cesarean birth may reach $3,500 or more.

To most families, these sums represent an enormous, if not intolerable, expense. And if inflation continues as it has for the past ten years, expect that these costs will double by 1987. How you handle such expenses depends on your financial picture—especially with regard to the amount and extent of your health insurance.

Group or individual policy?

Your health insurance may be a group plan or an individual policy, although most health insurance sold—85 percent according to the Health Insurance Institute—is sold to groups. If you are insured through your job or union, whether or not you yourself pay the premiums, you have group insurance. Its advantages over insurance purchased individually are:

• It is less costly (the employer may pay part or all of the premium).

• The benefits are much broader, and there are fewer restrictions, exclusions, and limitations.

• Your coverage cannot be canceled as long as you meet the eligibility requirements of the group (for example, active employment).

• You cannot be refused coverage.

The only drawback to group insurance is that you lose it when you no longer meet eligibility requirements—that is, when you quit work. This is a distinct problem for women who are planning to leave work when their babies are born, but who still want insurance coverage. Almost all group plans, however, have a *conversion privilege* that allows you to convert your group policy into an individual policy, usually within thirty days. It's a good idea to do this if you have no other coverage. But don't be surprised if the individual policy costs much more and pays much less. It may totally exclude coverages that were available under the group plan.

Some women who are enrolled in group insurance plans through their jobs are unsure whether they must work the full nine months of pregnancy to collect payment for maternity expenses. As long as eligibility requirements are maintained, the insurance company is satisfied and is not concerned with how far into your pregnancy you continue working. Eligibility always includes premium payments (if you take a leave, you may have to forward premiums to your employer). Eligibility *may* include full-time employment, in which case if you take a leave you may lose benefits. You should check this point with your personnel office.

In general, if you are offered a group plan through your job, take it. It is almost always a better buy than insurance purchased individually.

Your insurance policy

Most insurance policies provide coverage under three general areas—hospital, medical, and surgical—usually called *basic* benefits.

• Hospitalization benefits. Room, board, and nursing services may be covered completely, or you may receive a fixed amount— say, $50 a day—toward these expenses. Related costs, often called *ancillary expenses,* may also be completely or partially covered. These include diagnostic tests and medication you have in the hospital, and the use of special areas such as labor and delivery rooms. The anesthesiologist's charges may be considered an ancillary expense if s/he is an employee of the hospital.

• Medical benefits. These cover physician's services—for example, in-hospital visits (other than surgery). Sometimes, in-office and in-home visits are covered, too. Outpatient laboratory and diagnostic tests may also be reimbursable under this portion of your plan.

• Surgical benefits. These pay for the cost of surgical procedures. The amounts paid for various procedures are normally shown in the insurer's *surgical schedule,* a list of procedures and maximum payments. Sometimes, instead of a surgical schedule, the payments for doctors' charges will be based on a percentage (80 percent, 90 percent, 100 percent are most common). If your plan has full maternity benefits, both vaginal and cesarean births may be listed on the surgical schedule, along with the maximum amounts payable for each.

Everyone with health insurance has "basic" benefits. Unfortunately, as we shall see, basic benefits do not always cover maternity expenses.

Supplemental major medical protection is a form of insurance protection designed to help defray the costs of catastrophic bills. It is widely available, although you or your employer must pay extra for it. It also helps pay for any medical care *not* covered by your basic policy. Before you begin to receive major medical reimbursement you usually have to satisfy a deductible, an amount you must pay yourself. After that, major medical usually covers about 80 percent of all medical costs—in or out of the hospital. If you have major medical protection, it can come in handy when costly outpatient diagnostic tests, such as amniocentesis, are needed but are not covered by your basic plan. It can also be drawn on when you need special attention that requires frequent outpatient visits to your obstetrician—visits not covered by your basic plan.

Like the basic plans they are meant to supplement, many major medical plans exclude pregnancy.

Comprehensive major medical plans usually incorporate basic and supplemental benefits into one plan. Comprehensive coverage is usually available only to groups. And, again, they may exclude maternity expenses.

Maternity coverage

It would be great if basic, major medical, and comprehensive coverages always applied to maternity benefits. All too frequently, however, insurance companies have considered pregnancy a unique condition, one to which policyholders cannot apply their usual benefits. Often, "maternity benefits" are shown in a separate section of your policy or booklet. Many insurance companies have refused to cover maternity expenses at all, believing pregnancy and birth to be events for which families can plan and budget in advance. A 1978 survey by the Health Insurance Institute showed that almost half of the participants in new group policies had no maternity coverage.

Some insurers have seen the need for maternity benefits but have classed them separately. (In many cases, however, these distinctions are no longer legal—see the next section.) Before benefits are paid for maternity expenses, you may be required to be insured for a specified period of time (nine to ten months). Thus, if your coverage is effective, say, March 1 and your baby is born November 15, you may not receive benefits. This waiting period has denied many families coverage when policyholders have switched jobs or insurance companies in the middle of a pregnancy.

To further restrict benefits, some insurance companies have regulations that insureds cannot collect for maternity expenses the way they can collect for the expenses of illness or accident. For example, while Joe with a slipped disc found his hospital room and board completely reimbursable, Betty's maternity benefits consisted of one lump sum—anywhere from $175 to $500—that had to apply to everything: hospital room and board, physicians' fees, medications, tests, and any other costs Betty incurred. Even if Betty could have collected full hospital reimbursement, she might have found there was a four- or five-day limit on her hospital stay. Clearly, Joe with the slipped disc fared better.

Finally, many insurance companies have offered maternity benefits only with the costlier family option. Pregnant women who wanted the single option, either because they had no family or because the rest of the family was covered under another policy, could not collect maternity benefits under their policies. Sometimes the insured had to opt for a special maternity rider.

The 1978 amendment may affect your insurance

You now may have much better maternity benefits than ever before *if you are covered through group insurance by your employer.*

A recent amendment (signed into law on October 31, 1978) to Title VII of the 1964 Civil Rights Act prohibits discrimination in employment practices (including fringe benefits) on account of pregnancy. This law applies to employers of fifteen or more employees and requires them to be in compliance as of April 29, 1979.

After that date, employers could no longer offer fringe benefits—such as insurance—that paid less or different benefits for maternity than it paid for any other illness or accident.

Now, maternity benefits have been expanded for millions of women who are insured through their own or their husband's job-related health insurance plans *if* those plans are covered by the new amendment. Some of the advantages for these families:

• Maternity benefits cannot be excluded from health insurance plans—basic, major medical, or comprehensive.

• Pregnancy must be covered just as any illness is. As a result, those lump-sum or limited payments will disappear. If the plan pays full hospitalization for Joe's slipped disc, it must pay full hospitalization for Betty's maternity stay in the hospital. If the plan pays a certain percentage of Joe's in-office visits to his physician, it must pay the same for Betty's pre- and postnatal in-office visits. If diagnostic tests—such as Joe's outpatient X rays—are reimbursable, Betty's outpatient ultrasound must be, also. Cesarean surgery and simple deliveries will have to be included in each insurance company's surgical schedule.

• Wives of male employees cannot receive more comprehensive coverage than female employees.

• Single mothers will no longer face discrimination Because pregnancy must be covered just as an illness would be, women need not be married or enrolled in the family plan to collect maternity benefits. (*Note:* If you want insurance coverage for your newborn, the family plan may still be necessary.)

The new amendment is good news for the millions of women it covers. Before you rush out to collect your checks, however, remember that:

• This amendment applies only to employers and to the group insurance plans they completely or partially fund for their employees. This amendment has no bearing on policies you purchase on an individual basis or on policies you purchase from a club or social group.

• Your employer is exempt from the new law if s/he has fewer than fifteen employees.

• This amendment does not *force* your employer to provide health insurance. It says only that pregnant women must receive the same benefits as other employees. If no man receives a particular fringe benefit, such as health insurance, your employer need not provide it for you, just because you are pregnant.

Taking a close look

If your insurance is not affected by the 1978 amendment, don't panic. You may have adequate coverage even if your insurer is still covering pregnancy as if it were a special condition. Look carefully at the following:

• *Extent of coverage.* Be sure maternity benefits are provided at all. And be certain that costly complications, such as cesarean surgery or early hospitalization for toxemia, are covered, too, as well as hospital "extras," such as fetal monitoring and X-ray pelvimetry.

• *The waiting period.* If the policy is a new one, it may not cover costs of birth until nine or ten months have elapsed.

Individual or family coverage. You may have to opt for the more expensive family plan in order to get maternity benefits. And you may have to sign up *before* you get pregnant. If you are not married, you may have great difficulty securing maternity benefits.

Outpatient diagnostic tests. Amniocentesis, ultrasound, and stress tests are becoming almost routine, and each can cost in excess of $100. Will you be even partially reimbursed if your physician orders any of these exams?

And no matter what kind of insurance you have, you will want to consult the list of typical expenses on page 243, or obtain a list of similar costs from the hospital at which you will deliver, and measure your insurance against it. You'll then have a good idea of what your costs will be.

Coordination of benefits

Once you've deciphered the fine print on *your* insurance policy, you may not be finished. It's not unusual for women jobholders to be covered by two health insurance policies—their own and their husband's—if the husband, as is often the case, has a family policy. This does not mean that you can collect twice for maternity expenses. Group insurers frequently include a provision in their policies known as *coordination of benefits:* simply stated, you cannot collect more than 100 percent of your expenses. If the primary insurer (this may be the wife's or the husband's) pays, say, 80 percent of all covered maternity costs, the secondary insurer will pick up only the remaining 20 percent, regardless of its stated reimbursement. When applying for benefits, you deal first with the primary insurer, and then with the secondary one.

Couples who are paying premiums for two insurance policies should consider in advance the economics of this situation. If one of their policies covers close to 100 percent of expenses, the dollars spent toward maintaining a second policy may be wasted.

Newborn coverage

If the parents sometimes have too *much* insurance, there's one member of the family that often has none at all—the tiny newborn. If s/he is born with no problems, the costs may be manageable—say, $60 to $70 a day for nursery charges, plus the pediatrician's fees. If the baby is born with complications requiring surgery, intensive care, or costly medication, charges may run from

$700 to $800 a day over a period of weeks. Few families can handle such costs.

In the past—before about 1970—newborns were usually excluded from coverage during the first fourteen to thirty days of life. These, of course, are critical days for the preemie or for the baby born with congenital defects—days during which surgery and other intensive care may be most needed. Now, because of a campaign waged by the American Academy of Pediatrics, all but two states (Rhode Island and North Dakota, plus the District of Columbia) have passed laws making it illegal for insurance companies to exclude special care for newborns.

The problem is that policies written before the law was enacted can still exclude newborns. If your policy was purchased before the law was enacted in your state, you may find the fourteen- to thirty-day exclusion still in force. If your insurance originates in another state—say, where your employer's home office is located—the policy may conform to *that* state's law. You will have to read your policy carefully, pin down your personnel department or benefits officer, and perhaps even contact the commissioner of insurance in your state to find out what your baby's benefits include.

If special care for your newborn is not covered by your policy and you don't get more coverage, you are taking a big risk. More than two out of every one hundred newborns need intensive care.

Some insurance options for your newborn if you don't have coverage:

• First and foremost, look into family coverage to see if that option provides adequate newborn coverage.

• If you are with a group, contact the insurer and see if it will add the coverage. If not, you may be able to convince the insurer to add a rider to your individual policy to cover your newborn. For this privilege, you will have to pay extra.

• If you have "guaranteed-renewable" individual coverage, you may have to abandon the whole policy to make a change. Perhaps you, too, can obtain a rider, at additional cost, to cover your newborn.

Many policies do not cover *routine* newborn care. Others will pay nursery benefits under the mother's coverage, but only while she remains in the hospital. If she leaves and the newborn stays, the baby becomes a new patient and can be covered only if the parents have a family plan. Even then, the baby's charges may have to satisfy a new deductible.

Finally, remember that some insurers require that you notify them about a baby's birth by a certain time after the birth in order to claim benefits.

And you may want to know about . . .

• *Circumcision.* Usually appears on the insurer's schedule of surgical benefits, and is therefore reimbursable. If, however, the surgery is performed by someone other than a physician, it is not covered.

• *Miscarriage.* Under the 1978 Title VII amendment, miscarriage must be covered just as any illness or accident would be. Insurance policies not covered by the amendment may exclude benefits for miscarriage.

• *Private hospital room.* Rarely covered. Usually the cost of a semiprivate room is reimbursable and you must pay the difference between that and the cost of a private room. Amazingly, though, a private room may run only $5 to $10 more a day than a semiprivate room. The option is worth investigating.

• *Special meals.* Women who want kosher or vegetarian meals may have to make up the difference in cost between those and the regular meals offered by the hospital. Few insurance companies will pick up the tab for more costly fare.

• *Home health aides.* If professional nursing help when you get home is considered medically necessary, you may be able to recover part or all of the cost of hiring a home health aide. Before engaging someone, check your policy carefully or ask your insurance representative about this. Coverage may be available only if your physician orders the help, or if the help is licensed.

• *Certified nurse-midwife.* If your obstetrical caretaker is a certified nurse-midwife, you must check your coverage carefully; many insurance carriers are just beginning to delineate coverage for CNMs. Some policies still specify that only *physicians'* costs are reimbursable. Others will reimburse a CNM only if she is licensed by the state and working under or with a physician in private practice or in a certified hospital.

• *Home birth.* The only benefits payable would be for the physician's charges (up to the limits of the contract).

• *Alternative birthing centers.* Coverage depends on the insurance contract. Many contracts pay benefits to duly licensed and approved medical facilities only.

• *Health maintenance organizations.* HMOs are prepaid group health plans often offered through places of employment or through union membership. Enrolled members pay a fixed premium and in turn receive a wide variety of health services from a group of health professionals, some of whom are usually obstetrician-gynecologists. Expectant couples will find the following included in their coverage: complete obstetrical care, hospitalization and hospital services, laboratory tests, X rays, infant care, and sometimes medication. Occasionally an HMO will charge a nominal fee for prenatal visits ($1 to $2) and an extra fee for delivery. Members, of course, must use one of the physicians affiliated with or referred by the plan. Members are likewise limited to the plan's own facilities or affiliated hospital. Some HMOs have certified nurse-midwives on staff.

When you have questions

Insurance can be confusing. As you move through your pregnancy, accumulating bills, it helps to know exactly what your benefits are and how and when to get them.

The first thing you should do is look at your *certificate,* the employee's booklet of benefits. It should explain your coverage in broad terms. In the past, certificates have been pretty general, but insurers are now producing more comprehensive certificates. If yours is a newer one, it might just be detailed enough to answer your questions.

If it doesn't, try the benefits officer or personnel department at your office. Either will have a copy of the *master contract,* the formal agreement between the insurer and your employer. It lists all exclusions. Besides this document, you'll get expertise and advice. And if your personnel department or benefits officer is unable to answer your questions, s/he can contact the insurance representative, who in turn will refer to the insurer's *comprehensive manual.*

If you carry an individual policy, you should of course direct your questions to your own insurance representative. It may also be interesting and informative to speak with someone in the billing office of the hospital at which you will deliver. Employees there usually have extensive experience with a variety of insurers and may help explain to you not only the hospital costs but what is and what is not usually covered. They can give you a detailed accounting of what your hospital stay is likely to cost. And one of their credit counselors will probably be pleased to help you set up a payment plan so that you can meet your medical costs in good time and in good financial shape.

In addition, your physician's secretary or bookkeeper may also be an excellent resource if she is familiar with insurance.

Women who are preregistered at the hospital by their physicians may automatically receive, during pregnancy, a statement of charges that would attend a typical, uncomplicated birth. Sometimes a hospital will contact patients to request a deposit. Ask your physician if you have been preregistered—that is, if s/he has informed the hospital of your expected date of entry. If your physician has not done so, no matter what kind of insurance you have, *you* should be in touch with the hospital billing department as soon as you can. It's the only way you can figure out your expected costs and reimbursement. And as one hospital administrator pointed out, "The patient in trouble is the one who comes in and her doctor hasn't told us she's coming. Then she's socked with an eighteen-hundred-dollar bill."

CHAPTER SEVENTEEN
In the Hospital

Pregnancy is a life-style all its own. You wear a special wardrobe, adjust to new schedules, redirect your energies, and look at life a bit differently from before. Month by month you learn more and more about your body and how to deal with its changes. By the end of your pregnancy, your condition is like an old shoe—comfortable (at least emotionally!), familiar, and reassuring.

Labor and birth are a different story. If you had nineteen months instead of nine, you'd know little more about what a contraction feels like or what kind of experience birth is. Ten tours of the labor and delivery suite may help you memorize the floor plan but won't tell you how you'll *feel* in the hospital. Birth comes upon you quickly, and you don't have much time to familiarize yourself with the new sensations you're experiencing in a strange environment.

Of course, you do everything you can to prepare: read a lot, take childbirth-preparation classes, tour labor and delivery rooms. You ask questions—lots of them—of people whose opinions you trust. In this chapter, we're going to tackle some of the questions women ask most frequently about the hospital experience.

Labor

1. *What is the process of labor and delivery?*

Labor is the process by which a baby moves from the uterus to the world outside its mother. For most women, this process begins sometime between the thirty-eighth and forty-second weeks of pregnancy. It's not known exactly what causes the onset of labor, though some researchers think it has to do with an increase or decrease of certain hormones in the mother's body. Though there is a

254

wide variation in how long it takes, the average primigravida's labor lasts about fourteen hours, and the average multigravida's, about eight hours.

Before a baby can pass from the uterus, through the vagina, and out, the cervix (mouth of the uterus) must be effaced and dilated. This is accomplished by powerful uterine contractions. *Effacement* means the cervix, which is about two centimeters (three-fourths of an inch) long before labor begins, becomes shorter and thins out. *Dilitation* is the opening of the cervix to the ten centimeters (about the width of five fingers) necessary to allow the baby to pass through.

In some women, especially first-time mothers, effacement and dilatation may begin even before true labor starts. This is caused by painless uterine contractions—called Braxton-Hicks contractions—occurring late in pregnancy. Then, at some point, Braxton-

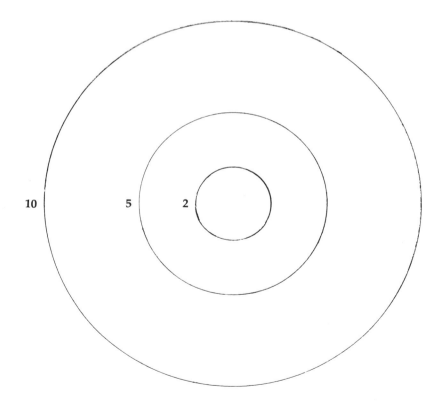

Fig. 15. Dilatation of the Cervix Shown in Centimeters

Fig. 16. Effacement and Dilatation of the Cervix

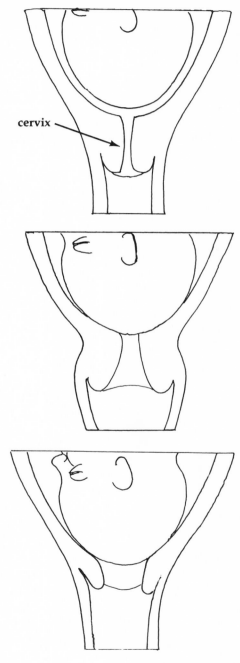

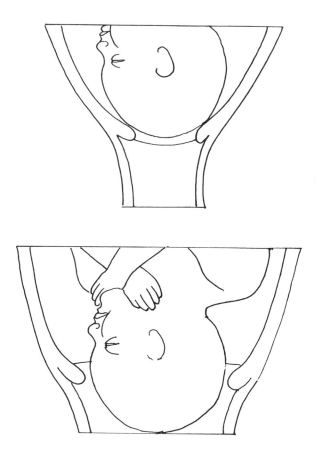

Hicks contractions become regular and painful, and come increasingly close together, indicating that true labor has begun.

Labor is divided into three stages. The *first stage* begins with the
first real labor contraction and ends when the cervix is dilated ten
centimeters. The first stage itself has three phases:

• *In early, or inactive, first-stage labor,* the cervix dilates to about four
centimeters. This is usually the longest part of labor, but it is also
the least painful. Contractions may be rather mild, five to twenty
minutes apart, and thirty to forty-five seconds in duration.

• *Active first-stage labor* involves dilatation of the cervix from four
to about eight centimeters. During active labor, contractions intensify, are three to five minutes apart, and last about one minute.

• *Transition,* when the cervix dilates from eight to ten centi-

Fig. 17.

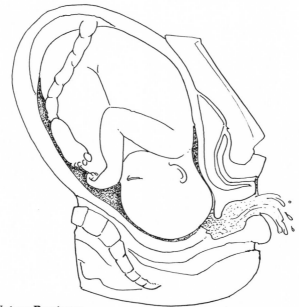

Bag of Waters Ruptures

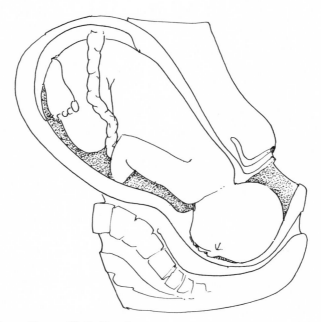

Baby Moves Down Birth Canal

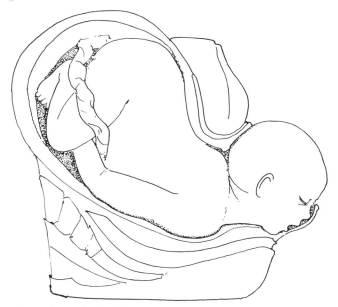

Crowning—Top of Head Visible

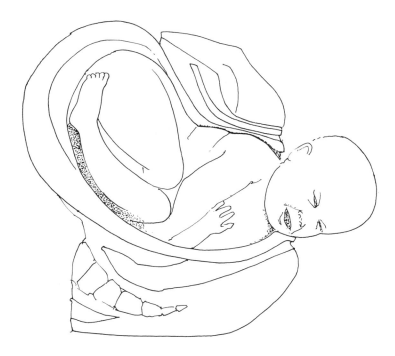

Birth

meters, is the hardest part of labor, but it is usually the shortest. Transition contractions are quite painful, about one to two minutes apart, and about ninety seconds long. During transition, many women experience irritability, disorientation, chills, nausea, vomiting, drowsiness, rectal pressure, "bloody show" (loss of the blood-flecked mucus plug of the cervix), and an urge to push the baby out.

When the cervix is dilated completely, the *second*, or *expulsive*, *stage* of labor begins. This stage, which lasts about a half hour to two hours, ends when the baby is delivered. Contractions are now farther apart and less intense than during transition. The mother feels an urge to bear down, which she can use to help push out her baby. When the baby's head finally "crowns" (begins to bulge through the vagina), the doctor may do an episiotomy (see page 272) to facilitate delivery. The head and then the shoulders of the baby are delivered, and the rest of the body quickly emerges. Shortly thereafter, the umbilical cord, which attaches the baby to the placenta, is cut.

The *third stage* of labor begins when the baby is born and ends when the placenta is delivered. Only a few contractions are needed to expel the placenta, and the third stage of labor generally takes no more than half an hour. After this, the physician will examine the placenta, and repair the episiotomy or any tears in the perineum.

2. *What should I pack for the hospital?*

Don't make a fetish out of your "hospital bag." The truth is, you'll need nothing more than a toothbrush, since the hospital can supply just about everything else, including gowns, paper slippers, sanitary napkins and belts, soap and towels, and even toothpaste. Many hospitals recommend that you leave your valuables at home. Nevertheless, you'll probably want to bring at least some of the following:

    toothbrush
    hard-soled slippers (the kind you don't have to bend down to
        put on)
    2 nursing bras (for those who plan to breast-feed)
    robe
    cosmetics and mirror
    hair dryer and hot curlers
    shampoo
    comb and brush

eyeglasses and contact lenses
books, magazines, needlework
pens and paper, birth announcements
address book
$5 to $10 in cash

Don't bring a lot of nightgowns unless you are sure you'll hate the hospital's, or unless you are very tall (hospital gowns will be uncomfortably short). After delivery, your breasts leak milk, you are still bleeding from the healing placental site, and you take your meals in bed. Unavoidably, gowns get soiled, so it's nice to be able to throw the one you are wearing in the *hospital* laundry. The snap shoulders make nursing easy, too. (That embarrassing slit in the back of hospital gowns can be covered if you wear two at a time— the second one front-to-back over the first.)

3. *How will I know when I'm in labor?*

Any of the following signs may indicate that labor—that is, regular, rhythmic contractions that will open the cervix and expel the baby—is about to start: (1) a ruptured bag of waters (you'll feel either a small trickle or a big gush of warm fluid); (2) "bloody show"; (3) an ache in the lower back or a crampy feeling in the groin.

Sometimes the regular, rhythmic contractions start with no warning. No matter how your labor begins, your physician or nurse-midwife will already have explained where and when s/he should be called, and at what point you should go to the hospital. Generally you call your birth attendant if: (1) the bag of waters has ruptured, or (2) you have established a pattern of regular contractions.

A primigravida may go the hospital when contractions have been five to seven minutes apart for one hour. A multigravida may be advised to leave for the hospital as soon as regular contractions begin, or when contractions are ten minutes apart.

4. *I've heard there's always a long registration hassle at the hospital, and that means a long separation from my husband. Is there any way to avoid this?*

Many hospitals now preregister maternity patients. Either the business office or the physician's office sends the woman, early in pregnancy, a form requesting the relevant information (name, address, insurance coverage, and so on), and when she returns it, she is registered. When the mother enters the hospital in labor, her partner need only report to the registration office and verify the information. The procedure could take as little as ten minutes.

More and more, hospital personnel are coming to recognize

the very important supportive role of the husband or partner, and are beginning to reduce the bureaucratic demands that separate parents. Some hospitals have established "mini"-registration desks right near the labor suite. In others, partners of mothers in active labor need not register at all until after the birth. Many big-city hospitals, recognizing the very real problems posed by automobile congestion, set aside temporary parking spaces for couples in labor.

Incidentally, if your hospital or physician has not preregistered you, call the hospital's business office and see if this can be arranged.

5. *Will my doctor meet me at the hospital as soon as I get there?*

Most of us would like very much to see a familiar face at the hospital, but whether you will or not depends on:

• *Your physician's schedule.* If you enter the hospital during your physician's office hours or while s/he is in surgery, you may have to wait a long while before s/he shows up at the labor room. If your physician alternates days on call with partners, you may be out of luck unless you go into labor when s/he is on duty.

• *Your physician's philosophy.* Some physicians don't see the point of hanging around during labor, reasoning that the nursing staff can keep them posted and lend valuable support to the laboring couple.

• *The hospital's personnel.* If the hospital has an Ob/Gyn resident on duty twenty-four hours a day, or a highly skilled nursing staff evaluating mothers who enter the labor rooms, the physician may not feel the need to report immediately to the hospital. However, the hospital will keep her/him apprised of your progress.

If you are in the care of a certified nurse-midwife, more likely than not you will have her or a partner with you throughout labor.

6. *I'm told that when I get to the hospital I'll have to sit in a wheelchair! Will they really treat me as if I were sick?*

It depends on the hospital. Some eschew the wheelchair routine because it gives laboring women a feeling of being ill or helpless; in those hospitals, wheelchairs are available only on request. At others they are customary, but if you'd rather walk, speak up.

7. *What does a labor room look like?*

You may labor in a private room, or in a room with two or three other women, with curtains separating the beds. If you do get private facilities (and at many hospitals there is nothing else), you'll probably find yourself entering an immaculate room about ten feet square, with an adjustable bed right in the middle and a comfortable chair to the side. A clock with a second hand will hang on the wall; it is there to help couples time contractions. Perhaps there will be a radio or piped-in music (some hospital labor rooms even have television). Large plastic bags on hooks or in drawers will hold your clothes and other belongings, a sphygmomanometer next to the bed will be used to read your blood pressure, and an IV apparatus will be wheeled to the bed. The gray metal machine with the blinking light, gently waving needle, and zigzag printout is the fetal monitor. It may or may not be in the labor room and may or may not be used, depending on the physician's orders. When it is hooked up, the laboring woman hears a regular *thud-thud* as the monitor graphs the strength of contractions and the baby's heartbeat.

Many labor rooms have private bathrooms stocked with towels, washcloths, soap, mouthwash, and tissues, and extra blankets, pillows, and ice chips are usually available for the asking. Often, labor-room lighting is adjustable, and there may be electrical outlets for those who wish to tape-record the labor experience, listen to cassettes, or play a radio. Photography may also be permitted in the labor room.

8. *If my labor and delivery are painful, and I don't think prepared-childbirth techniques are working for me, what kinds of medication are available?*

Obstetric pain relievers include *analgesics* and *anesthetics.* Analgesics raise your threshold of pain without making you unconscious. They help you relax between contractions, and blunt the actual pain. They are given during labor and may be administered orally, rectally, or by injection. Some common analgesics:

• *Narcotics.* Such narcotics as meperidine (Demerol) or alphaprodine (Nisentil), are frequently used for uncomfortable labors. They are injected, usually during active labor, and have the effect of dulling pain and inducing drowsiness.

• *Barbiturates.* Such barbiturates as Seconal or Nembutal do not relieve pain, they merely relieve anxiety. Usually, barbiturates are administered in the earliest stages of labor.

• *Tranquilizers.* Tranquilizers are given early in labor and, like barbiturates, are intended to relieve anxiety. Miltown and Valium are popular, and are often given in conjunction with pain-relieving narcotics.

Narcotics, barbiturates, and tranquilizers all cross the placenta.

By depressing the mother's system, they decrease the baby's oxygen supply. If the drugs are not given carefully, babies may be born groggy or unresponsive. They may remain so for several days.

Another kind of pain reliever you may encounter is the *amnesic* medication; probably the best known drug of this type is scopolamine. It induces a "twilight" sleep; pain is not inhibited, but after the medication wears off, the patient has no memory of it. Unfortunately, the patient has no memory of anything else, either, and the experience of birth is completely forgotten.

Anesthetics blot out all sensation, either by producing unconsciousness (general anesthesia) or by deadening nerves in a particular area of the body (local or regional anesthesia).

• **General anesthesia.** This may be injected or inhaled. Generally, it is administered very late in labor to diminish its depressive effects on the baby.

Local or regional anesthesia (also called *conduction anesthesia)* numbs specific areas by blocking impulses from the pain source to the brain. Locals are less likely to affect the fetus adversely, because little of the medication is absorbed into the mother's bloodstream. The locals include:

• **Spinal.** A single injection in the lower spine creates a numbing feeling from the point of injection down through the legs. Spinals are given at the time of delivery. They can slow down contractions and make it difficult for the woman to push the baby out. A frequent side effect of the spinal is a bad headache several days after birth.

• **Saddle block.** Also called a "low spinal," a saddle block numbs a more limited area than the spinal does; it affects only the part of the body that would touch the saddle if you were seated on a horse.

• **Epidural.** Applied continuously through a catheter inserted in the mother's lower back, the epidural causes numbing from the navel to the knee. Unlike the spinal, the epidural is not injected into the spinal canal.

• **Paracervical block.** The anesthetic agent is injected on either side of the cervix to diminish pain during active labor.

• *Pudendal block.* This deadens nerves around the vagina and perineum, and is primarily effective during the crowning of the baby's head.

• *Caudal block.* Like the epidural, the caudal is administered continuously through a catheter. It can be used effectively throughout labor and delivery.

All anesthetized mothers are continuously monitored. If anesthetics are not administered carefully, at the proper time, contractions may be slowed, the fetal heart rate may be diminished, and the mother's blood pressure may drop. After birth, the baby of an anesthetized mother may be sluggish or may have difficulty breathing.

Yet, the right anesthetic at the right time can be essential. It can give a discouraged woman a psychological boost or even a much-needed rest without depressing or harming the baby. Sometimes an anesthetic is a clear necessity, as when a general is administered to relax the uterus. The point is, every woman is unique and every labor is different. Your contractions may be painful, even though your best friend called hers "annoying." Her unmedicated labor may be inappropriate for you. Labor is no time for heroics; if you are truly uncomfortable, ask your physician for relief.

9. *Recently I've heard friends talking about "alternative birthing centers" and "early-labor rooms." What do these terms mean?*

Today, many hospitals have alternative birthing centers (ABCs), in addition to the traditional labor and delivery rooms. Basically, ABCs are for couples who want to have their babies in a homelike atmosphere but also want direct access to hospital technology and resources. Alternative birthing centers often consist of a lounge area, where women in early labor may spend time with their families and friends, and bedrooms, with rocking chairs, tables, stereos, plants, and a large, nonhospital bed where the baby is delivered. Couples are also encouraged to bring other items that will make them feel at home.

Women who wish to deliver in an ABC are carefully screened beforehand. Their pregnancies must be normal, and there must be no indication that labor and delivery will be unusual. During delivery in an ABC, the mother receives no medication and is not subjected to other hospital routines, such as shaving, enema, IV, and fetal monitor. If any problems arise, she is taken to the regular labor and delivery area. The new family stays in the ABC less than twenty-four hours before going home. A mother or baby who needs longer care is transferred to the regular postpartum room or nursery. Because of the shorter stay, total hospital costs are usually reduced for couples using the ABC.

Some hospitals that do not have ABCs have early-labor rooms. These are areas set up to accommodate women who arrive at the hospital in the early stages of labor and who do not need—or want—to be confined to bed. An early-labor room is similar to the lounge area of an ABC, with comfortable furniture, TV, radio, card tables, and so on. Couples can relax in an early-labor room until active labor starts and the mother is more comfortable in a regular labor bed. However, early-labor rooms may be used sporadically because, in many cases, expectant couples do not need to come to the hospital until active labor is under way.

10. *What is a fetal monitor?*

A fetal monitor is an electronic device that measures the fetal heart rate and the strength of uterine contractions during labor. It can alert the physician to signs of fetal distress. A skilled interpreter reading the monitor's patterns can often discern the reasons for the distress and initiate the appropriate medical response.

• *External fetal monitoring.* In external fetal monitoring, two straps are placed around the mother's abdomen—which many women find uncomfortable—to pick up the fetal heart tones and mother's contractions. These are transmitted to a small metal box, which graphs the measurements. The box has a vacillating needle and flashing light, and it emits a regular "thudding" sound. (When a laboring woman rests on her side—instead of sitting upright—this sound is often muffled.)

• *Internal fetal monitoring.* For internal fetal monitoring, a wire with an electrode that attaches to the baby's head or foot is inserted vaginally. The electrode picks up fetal heart tones and the mother's contractions, and transmits them to the monitor.

Some hospitals use external fetal monitoring for all their patients in labor. Internal fetal monitoring is usually done only in high-risk situations. Generally, internal fetal monitoring is considered more reliable than external fetal monitoring.

Some hospitals are experimenting with fetal monitoring by radiotelemetry, in which the laboring woman is not attached to a machine and can move about freely.

11. *What is "prepping"?*

Strictly speaking, "prepping" is the shaving of a woman's pubic hair before delivery. However, some people use the term to include all the preparation procedures a woman undergoes before she delivers. These include:

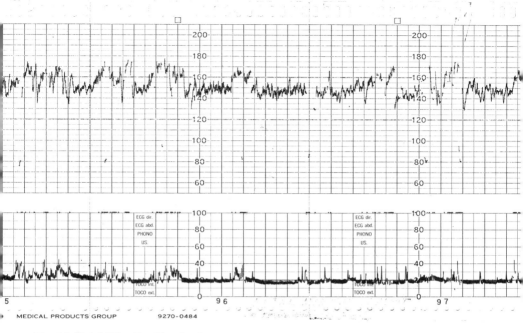

Fig. 18. Fetal Monitor Readout

• **Enema.** Unless labor is too far advanced, most hospitals prefer to give the laboring woman an enema. This empties the lower bowel and creates more room for the baby as it moves down the birth canal. Women have an enema early in labor to prevent liquid feces from being expelled when the baby is being born. After the enema is given, a woman in labor is usually told to stay on the toilet or bedpan until all fecal matter has been passed. The enema is an annoyance for most laboring women, and some even find it intensifies their contractions. If you feel strongly about not having an enema during labor, discuss this with your physician beforehand.

• **Shave.** The reasons usually cited for shaving pubic hair before delivery are that this procedure lessens the chance of infection and affords the doctor a better view of the birth area. However, some experts feel that shaving actually increases the risk of infection. Today, most hospitals favor the "mini-prep," which consists of shaving just around the vagina and anus, a procedure that takes less than a minute. The small amount of hair removed produces minimal discomfort as it grows back. In some hospitals, though, the full prep—the removal of all pubic hair—is still standard. In other hospitals, preps are optional and many patients choose not to have them.

•*IV.* Soon after most laboring women arrive at the hospital, they are hooked up to an intravenous (IV) drip. This is used to supply glucose solution, and, if necessary, analgesia and anesthesia, to the mother during labor, and to keep a vein open in case emergency medication is needed. Often, the IV apparatus is portable, so women in labor can continue to walk, if they wish, and to use the bathroom rather than a bedpan.

12. *Once I enter the hospital, do I have to stay in bed?*

Women in active labor usually feel more comfortable in a bed that they can raise or lower by pressing a button. But many hospitals permit—and even encourage—laboring women to get up periodically, move around, use the bathroom, and so on. Some experts feel that movement helps labor to progress more efficiently. Your mobility during labor may depend on whether you're attached to a portable IV.

13. *Besides prepping, what goes on in the labor room?*

When you first enter the labor room, a resident, nurse, or your own physician (if s/he is present) will perform a brief general exam and an internal exam to assess the progress of your labor. If your doctor is not present, the results of this exam will be relayed to her/him. Then a urine specimen will be taken and you may have an enema, shave, and IV. Periodically (at progressively shorter intervals) during labor, nurses will take your temperature, pulse, and blood pressure. They will also check fetal heart tones and the quality of your contractions. Your physician will do internal exams during labor, but infrequently, to reduce the chance of infection.

14. *Who will be permitted to stay with me in the labor room?*

Most U.S. hospitals allow *one* person to remain with the mother during her labor. This person may be the father of the child or a "significant other," (frequently the pregnant woman's mother). Some hospitals require that this person present a certificate stating that s/he has attended a childbirth education class. Other hospitals have no such requirement or do not usually enforce it.

Hospitals allow a partner for the laboring woman because they have come to recognize her need for support and encouragement. Also, women trained in certain childbirth methods need a partner during labor to assist them with various breathing techniques. In theory, the partner can stay with the mother for her entire labor, though sometimes the partner is asked to leave momentarily during prepping and internal exams. If couples do not wish to be separated, they should make this clear to the doctor or nursing staff. Some hospital personnel feel so strongly that the laboring couple should not be separated that they do not provide coffee or snacks that might distract the father from his role as labor coach.

15. *Is the labor-room staff trained in prepared-childbirth methods?*

Increasing numbers of women are relying on prepared-childbirth techniques to help them get through labor and delivery. Because of this trend, many hospitals require that their labor- and delivery-room staff be familiar with popular prepared-childbirth methods. This training is helpful when: (1) the laboring couple is separated (for example, during registration or prepping); (2) the father or partner cannot be present during labor; (3) the couple is having difficulty using the prepared-childbirth techniques; (4) the couple has never been trained in prepared-childbirth methods and may benefit from on-the-spot coaching.

Laboring women should not expect, though, that nurses will be able to coach them in breathing exercises for long periods. The length of time nurses can stay with a woman in labor depends on the total patient load and their other work responsibilities. However, a certified nurse-midwife will usually stay with her patient throughout labor and delivery.

16. *When and how will I be moved from the labor room to the delivery room?*

In a woman delivering her first child, the cervix must be fully dilated—to ten centimeters—before she is transferred from the labor room to the delivery room. Also, she may start the process of pushing out her baby in the labor room since this stage may take considerable time in a primigravida.

With her second or subsequent delivery, a woman may be taken to the delivery room when her cervix is seven to eight centimeters dilated, since delivery will probably proceed much more quickly for her than it will for a first-time mother.

Laboring women are usually transferred from the labor bed to a cart, which is wheeled into the delivery room. Then they are transferred again to the delivery table. Some hospitals, though, have transporting tables that are used as delivery tables, eliminating one uncomfortable maneuver for women in the late stages of labor.

17. *What is "induced" labor?*

Labor is induced, or started artificially, by administering drugs to the mother or by breaking her bag of waters. Induction is medically indicated when fetal or maternal health will be endangered if the pregnancy continues. But *elective induction* for the doctor's or patient's convenience has drawn much criticism in recent years. With induced labor there is the danger that the baby will be born prematurely if gestational age is not accurately determined, and then suffer a range of health problems. If not supervised, oxytocin, the drug used to induce labor, may produce such strong (titanic) contractions that the fetus may be deprived of oxygen or the uterus may rupture.

Delivery

1. *Who will be with me in the delivery room?*

Generally, the medical staff in the delivery room includes the attending physician, a nurse (or nurse-midwife, if available), and sometimes a nurse's aide or obstetric technician. If anesthesia is used, an anesthesiologist or nurse-anesthetist must be present. In a high-risk situation, a pediatrician usually attends the delivery. Other specialists may be called in if complications arise.

Many U.S. hospitals allow the father to accompany and stay with the mother during delivery, although often he must prove he's attended a childbirth-education class. In some hospitals, the mother may choose someone other than the father, or she may choose to have one person with her during labor and another person during delivery. Most physicians ask the attending father to stay behind or to the side of the mother's shoulders. A few, however, allow the father to come to the foot of the delivery table to have a better view of the birth, or even to help "catch" the baby.

2. *Some of my friends say they had "forceps deliveries." What does that mean?*

Forceps are instruments a doctor may use to help the mother deliver the baby. The instruments resemble tongs, or two spoons facing each other. In a forceps delivery, the physician reaches up the birth canal, fits the two forceps blades securely on either side of the baby's head, and then carefully guides the head through the birth opening. A woman is said to have a *low-* or *mid*-forceps delivery, depending on how far down the birth canal the baby's head has come before forceps must be applied. Forceps are indicated for deliveries when there is fetal distress or maternal problems that require a quick delivery. Forceps may be used to rotate a malpositioned baby, or to shift a baby to a roomier portion of the pelvis for a less traumatic delivery. When a woman has had a type of anesthesia that prevents her from pushing the baby herself, the physician usually employs forceps, and they are also used for premature babies, as a kind of helmet, to protect the soft head from excessive battering against the perineum. The *routine* use of forceps just to speed delivery has been criticized. Babies delivered with forceps may have slight marks where the instruments were applied, but there should be no permanent damage to baby or mother when forceps are used properly.

3. *What is a delivery table like? Will it be comfortable?*

In most hospitals, a woman delivers her baby on a narrow, waist-high table with leg stirrups to hold her legs wide apart. Today, women can often choose for themselves whether or not to use the stirrups.

The delivering mother usually lies on her back, with a pillow under her head. In some hospitals her wrists are strapped down, though nowadays this practice is increasingly unpopular among physicians and patients. Once the woman is in position, the table is broken, or its lower half removed, to allow the physician a better view of the birth.

Many women find the traditional flat-on-the-back (lithotomy) delivery position uncomfortable and hampering when they are trying to push the baby out. Some hospitals have adjustable tables or will provide pillows to place the mother in the more efficient semiupright position.

4. *What are Apgar scores?*

Most U.S. hospitals use the Apgar Scoring System to evaluate a newborn's condition both at one minute and at five minutes after birth. The baby's heart rate, respiratory effort, muscle tone, reflex irritability, and color are examined. Each of these five categories is scored, depending on how well or poorly the baby is doing. The highest score is 10, but most infants who are rated 7 or more are in excellent shape.

5. *Will I be able to see my baby being born?*

An adjustable mirror in the delivery room allows a mother the special thrill of watching her baby's birth. Today, many hospitals routinely make mirrors available, but couples should check before delivery to make sure the mirror will be in the delivery room and will be properly positioned.

6. *Will I be able to hold my baby right away?*

Many hospitals encourage immediate bonding between the newborn and its parents. Usually, if the mother wants and is able to, she can hold and even breast-feed her infant right after delivery. If the father is present, he, too, can have some time to hold his new son or daughter.

Before the mother goes to the recovery room and the baby to the nursery, the new family may enjoy about fifteen minutes of getting acquainted in a viewing area outside the delivery room, or they may all be able to stay together in the recovery room for the hour or so that the mother is monitored there.

7. *Will my husband be permitted to take photos or use a tape recorder in the delivery room?*

To remember the event better, some couples wish to take photos or record a tape during their baby's birth. Hospitals often permit cameras (no flash, though) and battery-operated sound equipment, as long as they do not interfere with the delivery. Some hospital administrators however, feel that picture-taking distracts the father from his vital support role during delivery, and so they discourage the practice.

8. *Where will I go from the delivery room?*

Depending on the hospital, a new mother may leave the delivery room and go to:

• A *viewing room* with her husband for bonding with the baby for about fifteen minutes. From the viewing room, she may go to the recovery room or directly to her hospital room.

• A *recovery room* for one or two hours. The father and baby may be allowed to accompany the mother to the recovery room, although some hospitals require that the father who wishes to do this must also have been present in the delivery room. In the recovery room, the mother's blood pressure, pulse, and temperature will be taken, and her uterus and the amount of vaginal bleeding will be checked. A baby in the recovery room is also carefully monitored, and if any problem arises, it is immediately taken to the nursery. Some recovery rooms have phones for the new parents to share their good news.

• *The assigned hospital room.*

9. *If I have an episiotomy, will it be painful?*

Most American physicians routinely perform an episiotomy just before the baby's head is delivered. An episiotomy is a cut in the mother's perineum—the area between the vagina and the anus—that makes the birth opening larger. To ensure that the incision and stitching will be painless, the doctor injects a local anesthetic into the perineum (unless the mother has already had a general or regional anesthetic).

However, most women experience discomfort for about one to two weeks after delivery as the incision heals. Some women are uncomfortable even longer. Hot baths, heat lamp treatments, and Kegel exercises may help relieve some of the soreness.

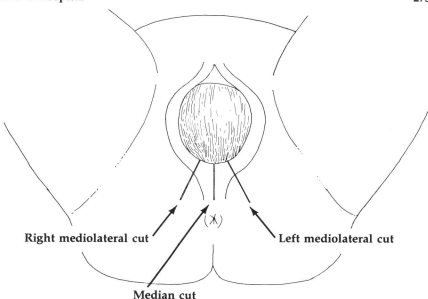

Right mediolateral cut   Left mediolateral cut

Median cut

Fig. 19. Episiotomy

Today, the episiotomy is a much-debated topic. Most physicians still feel the procedure is warranted to speed delivery and prevent perineal tears. But many women are asking their physicians to avoid doing an episiotomy if possible. They believe that training before labor and help during delivery may make the incision unnecessary.

Cesarean birth

1. *We are anticipating a cesarean birth. Will I have to go into the hospital the day before surgery, or can I check in that morning?*

Physicians often require the day-before check-in to ensure ample time for complete preoperative preparations: registration; signing of releases and consents; blood typing and matching; measurements of vital signs; shaving of the surgical area. Unfortunately, these procedures don't take very long, and far more time is spent waiting, missing your husband, and worrying about your children at home. You might discuss with your physician the possibility of entering the hospital the morning the birth is scheduled. In addition to the enema and catheterization, most tests can be done at that time. If your physician is concerned about the possibility of your eating (you must have an empty stomach for surgery), simply explain that you can refrain from eating at home just as reliably as you could in the hospital. And you'll probably get more rest at home, too.

2. *How long does the actual delivery take?*

From the first cut to the moment when the baby is gently pushed and pulled from the uterus, less than ten minutes may elapse. Speed is particularly important when general anesthesia is used; the faster the baby is lifted out, the less groggy it will be from the anesthesia. The greatest amount of time in the operating or delivery room is spent closing the several layers of incised tissue. This phase of birth may take about forty-five minutes. Following the birth, you will be taken to a recovery room, where you will be observed for several hours.

3. *I'm concerned about the scar. How big and where will it be?*

The scar you have on your *skin* following cesarean surgery may be a vertical line that runs from your navel to your pubic bone, or it may be a Pfannenstiel incision ("bikini cut")—a smile-shaped horizontal line just above your pubic bone and approximately four to six inches long. Many women prefer the bikini cut because it's almost impossible to detect once the pubic hair has grown back. You may be able to discuss your preferences with your physician. If yours is to be a repeat cesarean, though, it is likely the new incision will be made in the same place as the old one.

The incision you have on your *uterus* will likely be a lower-segment, or low-cervical, incision—a horizontal, smile-shaped cut across the lower portion of the uterus. The classical, or vertical, incision down the upper portion of the uterus is almost never made today, since the lower-segment incision is considered safer.

4. *May I have family-centered maternity care?*

If your hospital offers this option, you may take advantage of it. You may, however, want to adapt it to your needs: mothers who have experienced cesarean birth often need several days before assuming complete care of an infant. If you keep the baby in your room, depend on your husband to do most of the holding, changing for the first few days and cleaning (you can do the feeding). When he is not available, keep the baby in the nursery if you don't feel up to the responsibility. You may want to begin by seeing your baby during feedings only for the first few days. As you feel stronger and your own needs become less pressing, keep the baby with you for gradually longer periods each day.

FCMC is usually not rigid. You may care for your child as little or as much as you wish. The usually lengthy visiting hours for fathers mean that the work can be shared in the early days, when postoperative discomfort is greatest. Nurses are there to help and teach you. Above all, don't exhaust yourself. If you are comfortable and happy caring for your infant in your room, by all means do it. If you are tired and in pain, don't feel guilty or less motherly. Nap, rest, and relax. You'll have ample time at home to care for your baby!

Cesarean mothers, like others, should make a point of attending baby-care classes in the hospital.

5. *I'm going to have a cesarean, but I'm* not *looking forward to a solid week in the hospital. Can I leave early?*

Five to seven days is the usual length of stay for cesarean mothers, and all those days are needed by you to regain your strength. In the first days after surgery you will feel quite dependent and grateful for the nursing care, but as you recover you'll find yourself less thankful to the hospital staff and more eager to sleep in your own bed. At this point—whether it's the fifth, sixth, or seventh day—speak with your physician about checking out.

6. *Is there anything special to pack for a six-day hospital stay?*

First look at page 260 for the three-day list. Expand as needed. In addition, cesarean mothers who prefer to wear panties in the hospital should bring briefs, not bikinis (which can rub uncomfortably against the incision). Belts for sanitary napkins can be extremely irritating, and you may want to place soft, folded men's handkerchiefs between the belt and your incision, or use beltless sanitary napkins (have your husband bring a dozen or so from home if your hospital doesn't have them). As for footwear, some women say that wedged slippers are more comfortable than those with no heels.

7. *I plan to have a regional anesthetic for my next cesarean birth. Since I will be awake, I will want my husband with me. What are the chances of this?*

A cesarean is not simply surgery, it's also a birth. And many women want their partners to share the experience. Unfortunately, cesarean parents cannot always be together. State laws, city laws, hospital regulations, and physicians' biases all conspire to separate families. If your physician is a staunch opponent of the partner's presence during cesarean birth ("He'd make everyone nervous"; "He'd only faint"; "Why on earth would he want to see it?"), you have little hope of being together. If yours is an emergency cesarean, it is also unlikely that the baby's father will be permitted to accompany you. If your physician is enthusiastic about family-centered birth, find out what kind of arrangements you must make, or what kind of preparatory education might be helpful or required. And:

• Contact your local cesarean support group to find out about community laws and local hospital policies. Even an enthusiastic physician may be unable to buck a bureaucracy.

• Ask your hospital about pilot programs if it has no policy regarding a father's presence during a cesarean birth. Some administrators are willing to make judgments on a case-by-case basis, or would be amenable to an experimental program.

• Your physician may allow fathers in the delivery room in exceptional cases, or when s/he is simply made aware of the family's feelings and convictions.

Some women would like to see the actual surgery. If you are interested, ask for a mirror to be positioned for your viewing.

8. *What makes a physician decide on cesarean surgery?*
Common indications are:

• *Cephalopelvic disproportion (CPD).* In this situation, the infant's head is too large to pass through the mother's bony pelvis, and if surgery were not performed, the alternative could be a difficult and possibly dangerous forceps delivery.

• *Breech presentation* (feet or buttocks, instead of head, first). Some physicians routinely resort to surgery for breech babies of first-time mothers. Because the mother's pelvic outlet hasn't been "tested," these physicians feel it is safer to head off possible complications by turning to surgical methods. Others reason that surgery is less traumatic for the infant than the exaggerated twisting, pulling, and pressure that often accompany vaginal breech births. Routine "sectioning" for breech births is a hotly debated issue; its opponents urge that each case be judged individually.

• *Fetal distress.* Fetal distress occurs when the baby's oxygen supply is being diminished, and, consequently, its heartbeat slows or is irregular. This condition could be a result of compression of the umbilical cord, anesthetics, disease in the mother, prematurity of the infant, or separation of the placenta from the uterine wall. When fetal distress is present, the continuation of labor could be hazardous for the baby, and surgery may be indicated.

• *Failure to progress.* (also knows *dystocia* [dis-to'-shi-ah]). Despite regular contractions, the cervix may fail to open a full ten centimeters. In other cases, contractions may be too weak or irregular to open the cervix or expel the baby. If labor is prolonged, and labor-stimulating drugs prove ineffective, a cesarean may be the only or best solution.

• *Previous cesarean.* About half of all cesarean births are repeat procedures, simply because most physicians in this country believe, "Once a cesarean, always a cesarean." This assumption is now being questioned, and new studies indicate that a scar from a previous cesarean is not likely to rupture during a subsequent labor and vaginal delivery.

Postpartum

1. *I've heard that "afterpains" are worse than labor. Is this really true?*

More intense in multiparas than primiparas, afterpains are uterine contractions, lasting less than a minute, that may occur shortly after birth and continue for two or three days. These contractions enable your uterus to return to its prepregnancy state and to expel any remaining blood or pieces of placenta. Afterpains are often brought on by nursing. They are not usually worse than labor contractions, but are of the same intensity. To speed the return of the uterus to normal, you can gently massage the fundus or lie facedown with a pillow under your abdomen.

2. *What is family-centered maternity care?*

Hospitals implementing FCMC view the family as the most important unit in the birth experience. The health team and facilities are structured to provide support to the parents at every step of the childbearing process:

• Classes in birth and childrearing are offered.
• Tours of labor and delivery rooms are conducted.
• The staff knows about prepared-childbirth techniques.
• The father stays with the mother during labor, delivery, and, possibly, recovery.
• There are provisions for keeping the baby with the mother during the hospital stay.
• The father has extended visiting hours.
• There are provisions for sibling visitation.

Of all these, FCMC is most often associated with "rooming-in." In some hospitals, the baby remains with the mother twenty-four hours a day if the mother so requests. Elsewhere, rooming-in is limited to the mother's waking hours (for example, 9:00 A.M. to 9:00 P.M.). During this time, the mother is in charge of changing, feeding, and cleaning the infant (and will receive assistance if she needs it); the newborn is kept in a portable bassinet equipped with diapers, shirts, blankets, pins, cloths, and cleaning equipment. An important part of FCMC is flexibility. If at any time during the day the mother wishes to be alone, the baby goes to the nursery. The father may stay with his family all day and may even be able to have meals and snacks in the mother's room. During regular visiting hours, however, when others are present, the baby is returned to the nursery.

Rooming-in can be extremely satisfying for new parents who wish to become acquainted with their infant. With a supportive nursing staff, the experience can be educational for both parents. On the other hand, many second- and third-time mothers opt for minimal or no rooming-in (they see their babies at feedings) in order to get as much rest as possible.

3. *I have a two-and-a-half-year-old daughter whom I'll miss very much. Is there any way she'll be able to visit me in the hospital?*

Sibling visitation is the program you're looking for. Usually found in hospitals that foster FCMC, a sibling-visitation program allows little children to visit their mothers during the postpartum stay. Hospital rules vary: sometimes children over age six are allowed in the mother's room, and those younger must meet their mothers in a lounge or solarium. Sometimes siblings are actually allowed to hold their new brothers or sisters, either in the mother's room or in a separate viewing room. Some mothers consider sibling visitation so important that they will choose an obstetrician (and thus, a hospital) with this in mind.

An interesting variation on visitation programs is *grandparent* visitation. True, grandparents have always been able to visit the mother and gaze through the glass at the newborns, but in many hospitals grandparents are now permitted to hold and play with the new baby as well.

4. *How long will I have to stay in the hospital?*

An average hospital stay for a mother who has delivered vaginally is three days, although at some alternative birthing centers a twenty-four-hour-stay (or less) is customary if both mother and baby are well. Hospital checkout is authorized by your physician. If you prefer a longer stay than s/he usually prescribes, you should discuss your feelings openly. If you wish to leave the hospital earlier than is customary, you probably will have to speak with your obstetrician *and* the baby's physician. Many pediatricians think that a minimum of three days' observation is necessary for newborns. (If you do secure permission to leave the hospital earlier, you will receive special instructions concerning your baby's care at home.)

By the way, remember that hospitals, like hotels, have checkout times. If you leave after the prescribed hour, you'll be charged for the whole day.

5. *My sister complained that she didn't get any rest in the hospital because of all the interruptions. What happens exactly?*

Nursing care may seem intrusive at times, but try to remember that there are good reasons for postpartum routines. In the very best hospitals, sympathetic and flexible nurses minimize disruptions, but invariably they will have to:

- determine the tone of your uterus and ascertain whether it's returning to normal size
- check the amount and quality of your lochia (lo'-ki-ah), or bloody discharge
- take your temperature and pulse periodically (to check for infection)
- examine your breasts and nipples
- examine your episiotomy or cesarean stitches

6. *I don't know the first thing about infant care! I hope someone can teach me in the hospital.*

Someone will. All hospitals recognize their dual function as health-care provider and educational resource. Thus, it is well accepted that part of the nurse's job is to instruct new mothers in baby care. Some hospitals schedule daily classes with live demonstrations; others show filmstrips or videotapes on closed-circuit television. Some of the topics: breast-feeding, bottle-feeding and formula preparation, bathing the baby, as well as the mother's postpartum emotions, exercise, breast self-examination, and birth control. In some hospitals, all patients receive a handbook on baby and postpartum care.

7. *Will I have a roommate in the hospital?*

Hospitals usually have semiprivate and private rooms. Surprisingly, the private rooms may be only slightly more expensive. Most insurance companies will not reimburse you for the added costs of a private room unless it is medically necessary.

If cost is a factor, investigate the possibility of three- or four-bed wards, which some hospitals may offer.

CHAPTER EIGHTEEN
Postpartum Considerations

Pregnancy often seems like a long journey. For nine months a woman experiences many physical and emotional transitions. She eagerly anticipates reaching her destination: the birth of her child. But what about afterward? Can she resume the life she led before pregnancy? Is it true that nothing will ever be the same again?

During pregnancy it's hard to focus on the postpartum period—your life after the baby's birth. To begin with, you have so many more immediate decisions to make: which physician to use, where to have the baby, how long to work, what clothes and furnishings to buy, whether to breast- or bottle-feed. You'd rather savor the pleasures of pregnancy than worry about what will happen after the baby arrives. The postpartum period also lacks the drama associated with labor and delivery. And unless you've been through the whole process before, it's hard to understand exactly how much the baby will affect your life.

But since the postpartum period is a new and very different phase of life, you should try to plan for it and begin ahead of time to understand some of the changes you'll be undergoing. Some things to think about:

Your physical recovery

The immediate postpartum period can be a very demanding time, physically. The mother is recovering from pregnancy and birth—and surgery, too, if she's had a cesarean section. Both parents will probably be fatigued because of night feedings and the continual care newborns require. Now is the time for new parents to get help from parents, nurses, and housekeepers with tasks like cleaning, cooking, laundry, and errands. If you can't arrange for help, try to forget about everything but the essentials of getting through the day until you feel better and more rested. This may mean pickup meals, fewer visitors, and a less than spotless home for a while, but eventually the situation will improve. You and your partner might also work out a system whereby you alternate child care, so that each of you can have a specified time for rest. The point is to *expect* you'll feel tired, marshal all the help you can get, and not force yourself to be superhuman.

You may be depressed

Postpartum "blues" are probably the most often discussed aspect of life after the baby's arrival. The emotional "highs" of labor and delivery can give way to depression thereafter. You have nine months to get used to pregnancy, but almost overnight you are catapulted into the role of parent. New responsibilities, fatigue, discomfort from an episiotomy or cesarean birth, sore nipples, and afterpains can all contribute to a very discouraged, helpless feeling about your new role. On the other hand, the postpartum period can be a time of great joy as you discover the miracle that is your baby. Many new parents feel so fulfilled that nothing—even lack of sleep, dirty diapers, piles of laundry—can completely dampen their spirits.

It's best to realize that your emotions will probably fluctuate significantly during the immediate postpartum period, just as they did during pregnancy. One day you may feel quite organized and capable of being a terrific parent. You may enjoy the baby so much that the thought of being alone never enters your mind. Another day, everything may seem "out of sync," and the smallest tasks appear impossible. You may seriously question why you became a parent, and if it's worth all the work and worry. You may feel put upon by the burden of total responsibility for this new person and wish that you could return to your "pre-baby" existence.

One of the best ways to survive these ups and downs (and every new parent has them) is to talk with other parents, both new and experienced. These exchanges can help you understand that problems that appear so serious now are only temporary. Other parents can be sources of information or can offer much-needed emotional support. They can assure you you'll live through the colic, teething, diaper rash, and illnesses. Tap into other support systems now, too, such as family, church or synagogue, community or local women's groups, to help you get through this period. If your depression seems especially acute, seek professional help. It's difficult raising a child today. Parents, particularly new ones, need all the support they can muster.

You need time, too

Baby care can be time-consuming and involve many chores that are mundane, repetitive, and even unpleasant. Many new mothers, because they are usually the baby's primary caretaker, have trouble getting used to this aspect of their lives. Though you love your baby enormously, you may crave some intellectual stimulation, even if that only means reading a few pages of a book or having a moment of "adult" conversation with your mate. You may also lack time for grooming routines that used to be important to you. Again, things will get better as time goes on. But from the beginning of your life as a mother, you *must* have some time—however brief—to yourself. In the days right after delivery, this may mean just being able to style your hair, read a magazine article, or put on some makeup. Later on, it means making the time (and arranging for a sitter about whom you feel completely comfortable) so you can attend a lecture, play racquetball, have a manicure, go to an exercise class. Now and then, a brief respite from baby care can make a big difference in how you feel about your new role.

New ideas about sex

You may be one of those women whose sex life is relatively unchanged by childbirth. Indeed, some couples find they develop a special closeness after the birth of their baby, and that sex becomes more exciting. But other couples have difficulty getting back into their sexual routines. A number of things contribute to this problem: fatigue, physical discomfort, time-consuming child care, too many visitors. You may feel frustrated and resentful if sexual desires must be put aside because of other, baby-related concerns. Or you may feel that for the sake of your partner you *should* make love even though you don't really feel like doing so. Some women may have trouble feeling sexy if they think they are not as physically attractive as they used to be, or if they feel completely caught up in the responsibilities of motherhood.

During the postpartum period, try not to put too much pressure on yourself or your partner to "perform" sexually. Discuss your feelings (or lack thereof) with each other so that intimacy is maintained, even if sexual closeness is elusive. If possible, set aside some time to be alone together (easier with a first child than with a subsequent one). This can be during the baby's naps or after an early bedtime. You may feel like making love then, or you may just feel like holding one another and enjoying freedom from outside intrusions.

Deciding about your job

During pregnancy, you may have been certain you'd resume working after the baby's arrival. Now you're not so sure. Or you may have thought you were quitting work forever, but now wonder if it wouldn't be better, emotionally and financially, for you to go back to your job. After delivery, some women decide they really don't want to make the arrangements that will enable them to work. Or they may not feel happy about leaving the baby in someone else's care. On the other hand, some new mothers feel that returning to work will impose some order on their lives and offer them some much-needed time to themselves. And still other women return confidently to work, experiencing few problems in meshing career with motherhood.

Whatever your situation, whatever you decided about your job before you had your baby, you may feel different about it afterward. Sometimes, just delaying a return to work for a month or two beyond your original plans may be the solution. Eventually, though, you'll have to make a choice, weighing both your needs and those of your child.

To achieve a balance, many women modify their job arrangements—working at home or part-time, if possible, or on weekends or at night, when the baby can be left with its father or another family member, rather than a stranger.

If outside help is necessary, it's crucial that you feel comfortable with your choice of a caretaker. Ask people you trust about possible candidates. Sometimes a church or synagogue, community center, or senior citizens' group can refer you to a good sitter. Demand good recommendations and interview the sitter carefully. Have the sitter begin care for your infant while you are still at home to supervise and observe. Try to get a caretaker who will come to your home—it's less disruptive for the baby and will make getting to work easier for you. Make sure the sitter is well acquainted with your apartment or house and knows exactly what kind of care you expect. If the baby must be cared for outside your home, whether in a day-care center or private home, be sure you're comfortable with the environment and with the caretakers who will be providing love and stimulation for your child.

Combining work with parenthood can be made easier by sim-- plifying your daily routine. Try to get help with household chores, so that when you *are* home you can devote your attention to your family. Eliminate less essential activities, so that you don't feel you are spreading yourself too thin. Above all, try to structure your life carefully. You and your family can adapt and thrive if you all have certain unchangeable hours of togetherness.

Is it true nothing will ever be the same again? Unequivocally, yes. You will have new responsibilities that can at times seem overwhelming, and the freedom to come and go, or to have time just for yourself, will seem a wistful memory for many years. But you will also experience intense joy and pride, and discover, per- haps to your surprise, how unconditionally you can love another human being.

It's true: your job, your feelings about yourself and your part- ner, your thoughts and conversations, your house or apartment— all will change when your baby finally arrives. Yet the upheaval is a temporary one, for when you reach a new equilibrium, you will also have experienced great personal growth and a chance for joys unlike others you've ever known.

Acknowledgments

We were fortunate to have the assistance of many talented people while writing this book. We are deeply indebted to Martin N. Motew, M.D., and Jorge A. Valle, M.D. Their comments, suggestions, and commitment to this book were invaluable and are reflected throughout.

Many others took time from full schedules to answer questions or read portions of the text. Gail Barazani of the Art Hazards Project introduced us to the research on toxic substances and graciously lent her own unpublished material. Marilyn Miglin, president of Marilyn Miglin Model Makeup, Inc., Chicago, took time to discuss aspects of grooming during pregnancy with us. Arthur M. Osteen, Ph.D., of the American Medical Association, helped us understand professional distinctions; and Eugene Pergament, M.D., Ph.D., director of the Division of Medical Genetics of Michael Reese Hospital, Chicago, was kind enough to review and suggest material for our chapter on genetics and prenatal testing.

Harriette Foley of Marshall Field and Company was always gracious and warm in sharing her expertise gained from years of experience in maternity dressing. Nancy B. Meade, R.D., M.P.H., acted as our consultant on nutrition. She clarified for us the important issues in this complex field and was generous with her comments and ideas. Jacqueline Messite, M.D., consultant in occupational medicine, of the National Institute of Occupational Safety and Health, carefully read our section on occupational hazards in the workplace, as did Peggy Richardson of the Occupational Safety and Health Administration.

Chuck Hedke, director of product management of Blue Cross and Blue Shield, patiently guided us through the complexities of health insurance. Robert R. Mander of the American College of

Obstetricians and Gynecologists generously provided us with materials and was always available to answer our questions. Anca Pogany, associate director of nursing for obstetrics and gynecology at Michael Reese Hospital, and Pamela Shrock, childbirth educator, also read portions of the manuscript. Illustrator David Bruce Wolfe deserves special thanks for his medical illustrations.

If despite this generous assistance there are errors in the text, they are our own. We likewise take responsibility for all the material in this volume.

People in the following organizations responded expansively to our sometimes lengthy questions: the National Institute for Alcohol Abuse and Alcoholism; National Association of Parents and Professionals for Safe Alternatives in Childbirth; Center for Science in the Public Interest; American Dental Association; Health Insurance Institute; Action for Child Transportation Safety; American College of Nurse-Midwives; U.S. Consumer Product Safety Commission; National Institute of Occupational Safety and Health; Rachel Carson Trust; Art Hazards Project of the Center for Occupational Hazards; Home Opportunity for the Pregnancy Experience; Association for Childbirth at Home, International; Home Oriented Maternity Experience; The C-Section Experience (Chicago); C/SEC, Inc.; International Childbirth Education Association; La Leche League, International; Society for the Protection of the Unborn Through Nutrition (SPUN); The National Foundation–March of Dimes; Juvenile Products Manufacturers Association; Cosmetic, Toiletry, and Fragrance Association, Inc.; Occupational Safety and Health Administration.

Human rights agencies in all fifty states responded enthusiastically to our questionnaire about discrimination, and we thank those agencies for their assistance. Our lengthy discussions with hospital obstetrics administrators were invaluable in compiling our chapter "In the Hospital." We also appreciate the help of all the maternity shop personnel who gave freely of their time.

Finally, to the many women who completed our very detailed survey about pregnancy, and to those who let us tape-record their comments, go our special thanks. Their thoughts and suggestions comprise a significant portion of this book.

Bibliography

Among the hundreds of books, periodicals, pamphlets, and reports we consulted, the following sources may be of particular interest to expectant parents.

American College of Obstetricians and Gynecologists. *Assessment of Maternal Nutrition.* Chicago: American College of Obstetricians and Gynecologists, and American Dietetic Association, 1978.

————. *Standards for Ambulatory Obstetric Care.* Chicago: American College of Obstetricians and Gynecologists, 1977.

————. *Standards for Obstetric-Gynecologic Services.* Chicago: American College of Obstetricians and Gynecologists, 1974.

American Journal of Obstetrics and Gynecology. St. Louis: C. V. Mosby Co.

Apgar, Virginia, and Joan Beck. *Is My Baby All Right?* New York: Pocket Books, 1974.

Arms, Suzanne. *Immaculate Deception: A New Look at Women and Childbirth in America.* Boston: Houghton Mifflin Co., 1975; New York: Bantam Books, 1977.

Banet, Barbara, and Mary Lou Rozdilsky. *What Now? A Handbook for New Parents.* New York: Charles Scribner's Sons, 1975.

Barazani, Gail. *Safe Practices in the Arts and Crafts: A Studio Guide.* New York: College Art Association of America, 1978.

Bean, Constance A. *Labor and Delivery: An Observer's Diary; What You Should Know About Today's Childbirth.* Garden City, N.Y.: Doubleday & Co., 1977.

_____. *Methods of Childbirth: A Complete Guide to Childbirth Classes and the New Maternity Care.* Garden City, N.Y.: Doubleday & Co., 1972; Dolphin, 1974.

Benson, Ralph C. *Handbook of Obstetrics and Gynecology.* 5th ed. Los Altos, Calif.: Lange Medical Publications, 1974.

Berland, Theodore, and Alfred Seyler. *Your Children's Teeth: A Complete Dental Guide for Parents.* New York: Hawthorn Books, 1968.

Bing, Elisabeth. *Moving Through Pregnancy.* Indianapolis and New York: Bobbs-Merrill, 1975; Bantam Books, 1976.

_____. *Six Practical Lessons for an Easier Childbirth.* New York: Bantam Books, 1969.

_____, and Libby Colman. *Making Love During Pregnancy.* New York: Bantam Books, 1977.

Bingham, Eula, ed. *Proceedings—Conference on Women and the Workplace, June 17–19, 1976.* Society for Occupational and Environmental Health.

Birth and the Family Journal. Berkeley, Calif.: International Childbirth Education Association, and American Society for Psychoprophylaxis in Obstetrics.

Boston Children's Medical Center. *Pregnancy, Birth and the Newborn Baby.* New York: Delacorte Press, 1972.

Boston Women's Health Book Collective. *Our Bodies, Ourselves.* 2d ed. New York: Simon & Schuster, 1976.

Bradley, Robert A. *Husband-Coached Childbirth.* Rev. ed. New York: Harper & Row, 1974.

Brennan, Barbara, and Joan Rattner Heilman. *The Complete Book of Midwifery.* New York: E. P. Dutton and Co., 1977.

Brewer, Gail Sforza, and Tom Brewer. *What Every Pregnant Woman Should Know: The Truth About Diet and Drugs in Pregnancy.* New York: Random House, 1977.

Carson, Mary B., ed. *The Womanly Art of Breastfeeding.* Rev. ed. Franklin Park, Ill.: La Leche League International, 1963.

Chabon, Irwin. *Awake and Aware: Participating in Childbirth Through Psychoprophylaxis.* New York: Delacorte Press, 1974.

Colman, Arthur, and Libby Colman. *Pregnancy: The Psychological Experience.* New York: Herder & Herder, 1971.

Committee on Maternal Nutrition, National Research Council. *Maternal Nutrition and the Course of Pregnancy.* Washington, D.C.: National Academy of Sciences, 1970.

Consumer Reports, eds. *The Consumers Union Guide to Buying for Babies.* New York: Warner Books, 1975.

Davis, Adelle. *Let's Eat Right to Keep Fit.* Rev. ed. New York: Harcourt Brace Jovanovich, 1970; New American Library, 1970.

————. *Let's Have Healthy Children.* Expanded ed. New York: Harcourt Brace Jovanovich, 1972; New American Library, 1972.

Demarest, Robert J., and John J. Sciarra. *Conception, Birth and Contraception: A Visual Presentation.* New York: McGraw-Hill Book Co., 1976.

Dick-Read, Grantly. *Childbirth Without Fear: The Original Approach to Natural Childbirth.* 2d ed. New York: Harper & Row, 1959.

Dilfer, Carol S. *Your Baby, Your Body.* New York: Crown Publishers, 1977.

Donovan, Bonnie. *The Cesarean Birth Experience: A Practical, Comprehensive, and Reassuring Guide for Parents and Professionals.* Boston: Beacon Press, 1978.

Eiger, Marvin S., and Sally W. Olds. *The Complete Book of Breastfeeding.* New York: Workman Publishing Co., 1972; Bantam Books, 1973.

Epstein, Samuel. *The Politics of Cancer.* San Francisco: Sierra Club Books, 1978.

Ewy, Donna, and Rodger Ewy. *Preparation for Childbirth: A Lamaze Guide.* Rev. ed. Boulder, Colo.: Pruett Publishing Co., 1976.

Gamper, Margaret. *Preparation for the Heir-Minded.* Hammond, Ind.: Sheffield Press, 1977.

Guttmacher, Alan F. *Pregnancy, Birth and Family Planning: A Guide for Expectant Parents in the 1970s.* New York: Viking Press, 1973.

Hausknecht, Richard, and Joan Rattner Heilman. *Having a Cesarean Baby.* New York: E. P. Dutton and Co., 1978.

Hazell, Lester D. *Commonsense Childbirth.* New York: G. P. Putnam's Sons, 1969; Berkley Publishing Corp., 1976.

Hunt, Vilma R. *Occupational Health Problems of Pregnant Women.* Washington, D.C.: U.S. Department of Health, Education and Welfare, 1975.

Ingelman-Sundberg, Axel, and Claes Wirsén. *A Child Is Born: The Drama of Life Before Birth.* New York: Delacorte Press, 1966.

Journal of Pediatrics. St. Louis: C. V. Mosby Co.

Journal of the American Medical Association. Chicago: American Medical Association.

Karmel, Marjorie. *Thank You, Dr. Lamaze.* Philadelphia: J. B. Lippincott Co., 1959.

Kitzinger, Sheila. *The Experience of Childbirth.* Taplinger Publishing Co., 1972; 4th rev. ed., Penguin Books, 1978.

———. *Giving Birth: The Parents' Emotions in Childbirth.* New York: Taplinger Publishing Co., 1971; Schocken Books, 1978.

Klaus, Marshall H., and John H. Kennell. *Maternal-Infant Bonding: The Impact of Early Separation or Loss on Family Development.* St. Louis: C. V. Mosby Co., 1976.

Lang, Raven. *Birth Book.* Palo Alto, Calif.: Science & Behavior Books, 1972.

Lappé, Frances Moore. *Diet for a Small Planet.* Rev. ed. New York: Ballantine Books, 1975.

Laws, Priscilla. *X-Rays: More Harm Than Good?* Emmaus, Pa.: Rodale Press, 1977.

Leboyer, Frederick. *Birth Without Violence.* New York: Alfred A. Knopf, 1975.

Maternal and Child Health Unit, California Department of Health. *Nutrition During Pregnancy and Lactation.* Sacramento: California Department of Health, 1978.

Messite, Jacqueline, and M. Bond. "Considerations for Women and Work," in C. Zenz, ed., *Occupational Medicine,* Vol. II Forthcoming.

Moss, Stephen J. *Your Child's Teeth: A Parent's Guide to Making and Keeping Them Perfect.* Boston: Houghton Mifflin Co., 1977.

National Institute for Occupational Safety and Health, and American College of Obstetricians and Gynecologists. *Comprehensive Bib-*

liography on Pregnancy and Work. Rockville, Md.: National Institute for Occupational Safety and Health, U.S. Department of Health, Education and Welfare, 1978.

————. Guidelines on Pregnancy and Work. Rockville, Md.: National Institute for Occupational Safety and Health, U.S. Department of Health, Education and Welfare, 1977.

Noble, Elizabeth. Essential Exercises for the Childbearing Year: A Guide to Health and Comfort Before and After Your Baby Is Born. Boston: Houghton Mifflin Co., 1976.

Null, Gary, and Steve Null. Protein for Vegetarians. New York: Pyramid Books, 1974.

Pediatrics. Evanston, Ill.: American Academy of Pediatrics.

Preventive Medicine. New York: Academic Press.

Pryor, Karen. Nursing Your Baby. Rev. ed. New York: Harper & Row, 1973; Pocket Books, 1977.

Richardson, Stephen A., and Alan Guttmacher, eds. Childbearing: Its Social and Psychological Aspects. Baltimore: Williams & Wilkins Co., 1967.

Robinson, Corinne Hogden. Fundamentals of Normal Nutrition. 2d ed. New York: Macmillan, 1973.

Rugh, Roberts, et al. From Conception to Birth: The Drama of Life's Beginnings. New York: Harper & Row, 1971.

Simkin, Penny. NAPSAC Directory of Alternative Birth Services. Marble Hill, Mo.: National Association of Parents and Professionals for Safe Alternatives in Childbirth, 1978.

Spock, Benjamin. Baby and Child Care. Rev. ed. New York: Hawthorn Books, 1968; Pocket Books, 1976.

Stellman, Jeanne Mager. Women's Work, Women's Health: Myths and Realities. New York: Pantheon Books, 1978.

Stewart, David, and Lee Stewart. Safe Alternatives in Childbirth. 2d ed. Marble Hill, Mo.: National Association of Parents and Professionals for Safe Alternatives in Childbirth, 1977.

————,eds. Twenty-first Century Obstetrics Now! 2d ed. 2 vols. Marble Hill, Mo.: National Association of Parents and Professionals for Safe Alternatives in Childbirth, 1978.

U.S. Consumer Product Safety Commission. *It Hurts When They Cry.* Washington, D.C.: U.S. Consumer Product Safety Commission, 1976.

Vellay, Pierre. *Childbirth Without Pain.* New York: E. P. Dutton Co., 1960.

Ward, Charlotte, and Fred Ward. *The Home Birth Book.* Washington, D.C.: Inscape Publishers, 1976.

Wertz, Richard W., and Dorothy C. Wertz. *Lying-In: A History of Childbirth in America.* New York: Free Press, 1977.

Williams, John Whitridge. *Obstetrics.* Edited by Louis M. Hellman *et al.* 14th ed. New York: Appleton-Century-Crofts, 1971.

Wright, Erna. *The New Childbirth.* New York: Hart Publishing Co., 1968.

Index